Anxiety Disorder Explained

Anxiety Disorder Types, Diagnosis, Symptoms,
Treatment, Causes,
Neurocognitive Disorders, Prognosis, Research,
History, Myths, and More!

By Frederick Earlstein

Foreword

Fear and anxiety may be unpleasant emotions or experiences, but they do serve a useful function in a person's life – such feelings bring a rush of adrenaline and prepare a person's body for immediate action when there is some impending threat or danger.

However, when there is no significant or appreciable danger in the immediate vicinity, and by all accounts the fear and anxiety that one is experiencing is illogical and irrational, then such an experience becomes more disruptive and useful. When it happens repeatedly and over a long period of time, it becomes debilitating and restrictive to one's quality of life. Thus, it becomes properly classified as an Anxiety Disorder.

In this book, we explore the different types of Anxiety Disorders, the signs and symptoms, possible causes, and the various treatments now available.

Table of Contents

Introduction

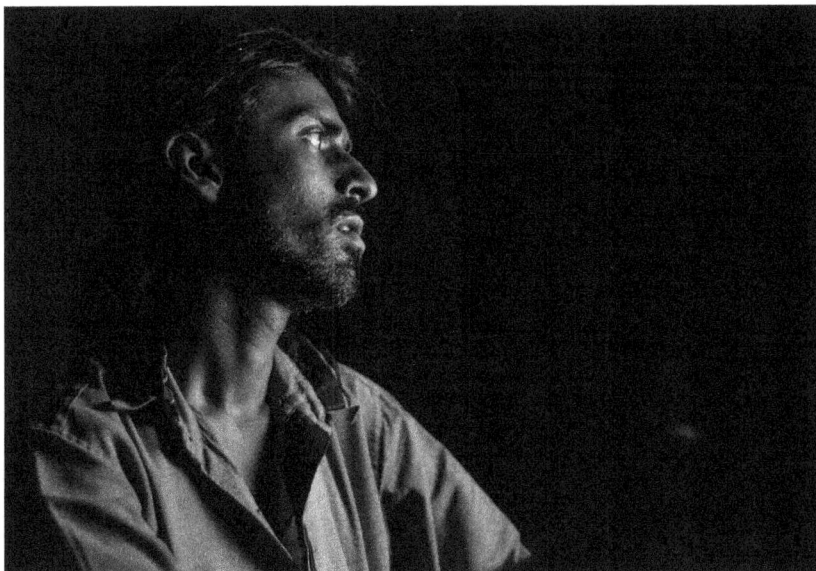

Anxiety Disorders have been part of the human experience for as long as we can remember – and written records have recognized by various names throughout the centuries. It wasn't until recent years, however, that it was properly recognized as a mental disorder that requires medical diagnosis and treatment. Today, Anxiety Disorder is one of the most prevalent psychological conditions in the world today, and also one of the most undiagnosed and untreated.

The good news is that Anxiety Disorders are mostly treatable, and a combination of pharmacological and psychotherapeutic treatments have had great success in helping people conquer their anxieties or otherwise develop better coping strategies that enable them to live a better quality of life.

Indeed, one of the characteristics of Anxiety Disorders are how intrusive they can be to a person's normal, day-to-day existence. The persistent and recurring fears, worries, and terror that one experiences during an episode of an anxiety disorder can cause them to voluntarily limit their reach in their environment, thus preventing them from creating social relationships, exploring the opportunities around them, or finding room for personal growth and development.

Important Terms to Know

Addiction – uncontrollable craving or desire for something

Adrenaline – i.e., epinephrine, a hormone produced by the adrenal gland causing symptoms experienced during moments of fear, worry, panic, or during threatening and stressful situations. Its function is to prepare the body for immediate action during emergency situations.

Agoraphobia – fear of being in public places

Anticonvulsant – drugs used to treat epileptic seizures

Antidepressant medication – drugs or medication used to treat depression, e.g., SSRIs and SNRIs

Anxiety – feeling of apprehension, worry, fear, or dread. Anxiety is considered normal unless the symptoms become excessive, in which case it is classified as an Anxiety Disorder

Anxiety Disorder – a group of psychiatric disorders characterized by excessive anxiety

Asthma – lung disorder characterized by inflammation that leads to breathing difficulties

Avoidance – tendency to stay away from places, individuals, or thoughts that cause or remind one of stressful or a traumatic experience

Behavioral Therapy – treatment involving the management of problematic behaviors

Benzodiazepines – minor tranquilizing agents

Binge eating – compulsive consumption of excessive quantities of food

Chronic – continuing or recurring condition with persistent symptoms

Cognitive – related to thoughts or intellectual activity

Cognitive Behavioral Therapy (CBT) – form of psychotherapy where a patient learns to identify negative thought patterns and are thought modifying or coping behaviors and strategies

Comorbid – Disorders that co-occur with another mental or physical disorder

Complementary Treatment – Outside mainstream medical practice, treatments that may be administered by practitioners in homeopathy, acupuncturists, etc.

Compulsion – repetitive and uncontrollable urge to perform certain activities or rituals, often accompanied by considerable anxiety

Depersonalization – a feeling of strangeness or unreality to oneself

Depression – mood characterized by loss of energy and interest in pleasurable things, feelings of worthlessness, and sometimes recurrent thoughts of death or suicide

Depressive episode – period of depressed mood

Diagnosis – defining a disorder through a set of signs and symptoms, and based on specific standards or criteria

Dopamine – brain chemical or neurotransmitter whose low levels seem to contribute to depression

Dysthmia – i.e., dysthymic disorder; mood disorder related to depression

Endorphins – chemical substance in the brain that reduces or blocks pain perception

Exposure Therapy – therapy that aims to expose the patient to the source of anxiety, where worry or anxiety reactions are addressed

Generalized Anxiety Disorder (GAD) – type of Anxiety Disorder characterized by worry over daily things

Grief – Normal emotional reaction to loss

Hot flashes – sudden wave of body heat caused by hormonal changes

Hypothyroidism – condition in which the thyroid gland does not produce enough hormones, may lead to fatigue, weight gain, or depression

Insomnia – inability to sleep

Learning disorder – disorder where an individual has difficulty learning basic or primary skills such as reading, writing and arithmetic

Mania – mood characterized by an abnormal and persistent elevated mood and hyperactivity

Melancholy – involves symptoms usually characteristic of depression

Mood disorder – disorder characterized by persistent mood disruptions, whether depressive or elevated mood

Neurotransmitters – brain chemicals travelling from neuron to nerve cells that constitute brain signals between cells

Obsession – intrusive and persistent thought, desire, or preoccupation

Obsessive Compulsive Disorder (OCD) – mood disorder characterized by repetitive rituals in order to decrease anxiety

Oppositional defiant disorder – disorder characterized by persistent and age-inappropriate defiant behavior

Palpitations – strong, rapid heartbeat and a feeling that your heart is about to burst out of your chest

Panic attack – sudden, unexpected and intense attack of anxiety accompanied by physical symptoms that builds to a peak within 10 minutes, generally subsiding within 30 minutes

Panic disorder – anxiety disorder comprised of repetitive and debilitating panic attacks

Paranoia – delusional perception that there are real or imagined threats against you or those close to you

Phobia – persistent and irrational fear of a specific object, environment or situation

Post-traumatic Stress Disorder – i.e., PTSD, this condition usually takes place after a person experiences a traumatic event.

Prognosis – clinical prediction of a disorder over time

Psychiatric disorder – disorder affecting one's cognitive, behavioral and emotional functions

Psychosis – a disorder that causes personality disintegration and a loss of contact with reality

Psychotherapy – a method of treatment characterized by helping people change their approach to situations or objects that otherwise cause them anxiety or distress

Recurrence – when an attack or episode takes place again after what seemed to be effective treatment

Relapse – reappearance of symptoms after the patient has believed to respond positively to treatment

Sedative – medication that induces relaxation and sleep

Selective mutism – disorder characterized by the inability to speak in certain settings or around unfamiliar people

Separation anxiety disorder – excessive anxiety related to the separation from something to which an individual is strongly attached; e.g., a child leaving home and going to school for the first time

Serotonin – a neurotransmitter that is linked to depression

Selective Serotonin Reuptake Inhibitors (SSRIs) – drugs intended to inhibit the reuptake of serotonin

Side effects – effects of drugs that may be favourable or unfavourable, and which are additional to the desired effects

Social Phobia – a fear of unfamiliar people or situations, or those involving social interaction and being the center of attention

Substance abuse – unhealthy and excessive use of substances that are usually illegal

Trigger – something that sets off or stimulates an expected response, or a predisposing event

Withdrawal – symptoms that occur when addictive drugs or substances are abruptly discontinued

Chapter One: What is an Anxiety Disorder

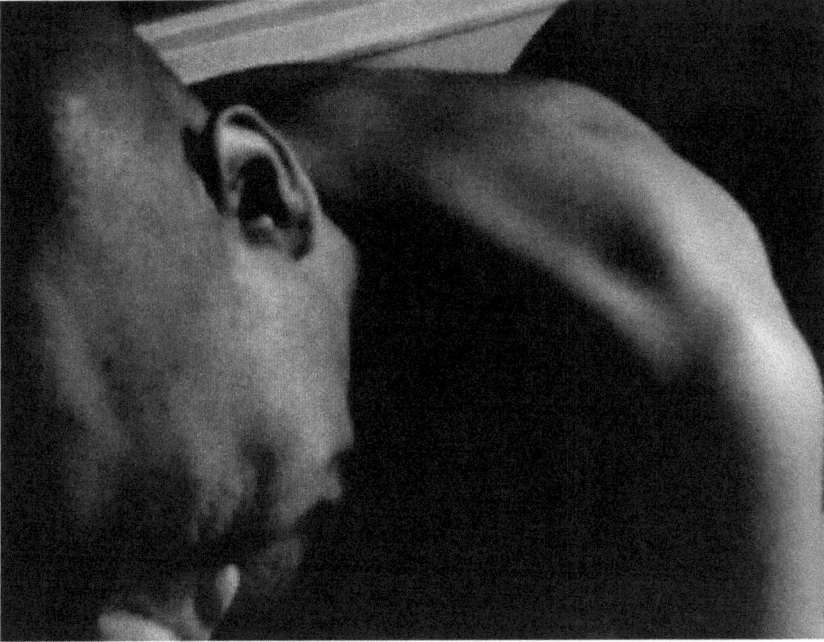

While it is true that anxiety as a human emotion is a normal, albeit temporary, part of life, it can sometimes happen that the feeling of anxiety is not temporary, but long-term. Anxiety can be appropriate in certain instances, but if it happens too regularly, or if it lasts for too long a time, then its consequences can become quite severe. When this happens, a person can be said to suffer from an anxiety disorder.

Being a long-term condition, an anxiety disorder can interfere with much of a person's life, including one's job or school performance and social relationships. It can interfere with one's capacity to live a normal life to the extent that it becomes considered as a serious mental illness requiring appropriate diagnosis and treatment.

Anxiety disorders are now considered to be one of the most common types of psychiatric disorders, and are often experienced with tangible physical symptoms such as fatigue, concentration problems, irritability, a fast heart rate, shakiness, restlessness, muscular tension, and sleep disturbances. Rather unfortunately, however, this widely prevalent condition is also one of the most under-recognized and under-treated clinical problems in the world.

Defining Anxiety Disorder

If you take the worries that you experience with normal feelings of anxiety, prolong it, which effectively only worsens the effects of those worries, then you have an anxiety disorder.

There are different types of Anxiety Disorders, and these are all properly classified as mental disorders characterized primarily by a feeling of excessive, persistent, and chronic worry, anxiety, or fear.

It is considered a disorder because the effects, regardless of which type it is, are intrusive enough that it interferes with a person's ability to live a normal life. Because of such intrusive and excessive thoughts, worries or concerns, a person either avoids the events or situations that trigger such emotions, isolates himself or herself, or otherwise turns to unhealthy means of coping with the anxiety such as aggression, substance abuse, or repression.

Almost everyone is expected to suffer from some form of anxiety during the course of one's life, particularly during stressful or traumatic experiences. It isn't precisely certain why some people are unable to move past such periods of intense anxiety, and why their experiences grow to become Anxiety Disorders, but it is suspected that the cause can be traced to a unique combination of genetic and environmental factors. It is also suspected that many people who have Anxiety Disorders go for a long time without being properly diagnosed and treated. One of the best ways to provide people with the means and strategies of better coping with the symptoms they experience is to spread awareness of this condition.

Myths about Anxiety Disorders

Perhaps because it is classified as a mental illness, or because (albeit in a less intense and pervasive way) everybody has suffered from anxiety at one point or another in their lives, Anxiety Disorders have been rife with myths and misconceptions – from not being a real illness, to methods of treatment and how to cope, and how it reflects upon the person suffering from the Anxiety Disorder. Yes, there does seem to be a stigma attached to mental disorders in general, and also to Anxiety Disorders in particular. But much of it is really rooted in the lack of public or general information about this condition which has since been recognized by the medical world as a valid condition that needs appropriate diagnosis and treatment, just like any illness or condition.

In this section, we take a look at some of the more common myths surrounding Anxiety Disorders, not only in an effort to spread information and educate the public about Anxiety Disorders, but also to validate the very real and tangible symptoms that a person with an Anxiety Disorder suffers from.

- *That only nervous, weak, or illogical people suffer from Anxiety Disorders.*

Everyone is prone to suffering from anxiety at one point or another in their lives. It is currently the most common condition affecting people all over the world, and it can affect both men and women equally. After all, everybody suffers from stressful situations, and everybody has some fear or something that they are anxious about, and at certain moments, those fears or worries can grow all out of proportion, thus paving the way for anxiety attacks. Phobias, for instance, are quite common, it doesn't take any personal weakness or characteristic nervousness in a person to suffer from what are essentially irrational fears.

And the truth is that persons suffering from Anxiety Disorders often do realize that their fears are irrational. They are no less intelligent, competent, or capable than anyone else, but an anxiety attack can and often does affect one's ability to function, and logic or rationality will often not help when one is in the grip of an anxiety attack. Again, validation and appropriate treatment methods are far more helpful in the long run than a simple and often curt dismissal of the very real symptoms of this condition.

- *That if a panic attack gets too bad, you can pass out, faint, lose control, or have a heart attack.*

Fainting or passing out comes about due to a sudden drop in temperature, and this is unlikely to happen during a panic attack because your blood pressure, instead of falling, actually rises slightly. Neither is a person in imminent danger of a heart attack, even though it might feel that way with the rapid increase in one's heartbeat.

Sometimes things are not necessarily as bad as we fear them to be, and this includes the possible effects of having a panic attack. Most times, such situations only get worse because we anticipate the worst. While the physical and emotional symptoms of a panic attack are quite real, simply knowing and remembering that such attacks can be ridden out without any deleterious and long-lasting effects can be one effective method of coping with the condition.

- *That tranquilizers and sleeping pills are the best treatment for anxiety.*

Helpful as they may often be, medication is only one part of a comprehensive treatment for Anxiety Disorders.

Their effects are only temporary, after all, and does not guarantee any long-lasting relief. In addition, too much use can also cause addiction and dependence, which in the long run would be far more detrimental to the person than suffering from anxiety attacks alone.

Many medical professionals now recommend a more comprehensive way of treating Anxiety Disorders, and while medication such as tranquilizers and sleeping pills do have their place, other methods like recommended exercises and therapies should also be pursued. In many instances, Anxiety Disorders such as phobias can, with the proper approach, be overcome.

- *That anxiety attacks are just excessive worrying, and a person should just pull himself/herself together because the feeling will soon pass.*

While everyone experiences moments of worries and fears, for a person suffering from an Anxiety Disorder, the feeling is excessive, uncontrollable, acute, and will not simply disappear. In fact, there is often no trigger at all for the onset of panic attacks. The very unpredictability and often disproportionate sensations and feelings caused by such an attack, even if a person does strive to manage life's challenges well enough, argues against simply dismissing this condition as something that is simply part of normal life that will soon pass, or something that should either be ignored or conquered by will power alone.

The healthier option is to recognize the very real nature and symptoms of this condition, get a proper diagnosis, and proactively address it with recommended treatments and therapies.

- *That it isn't real, or that it is all in your head.*

People who actually do suffer from Anxiety Disorders will beg to disagree, and with good reason. Part of what characterizes Anxiety Disorders – in addition to the difficulties caused by its unpredictability and oftentimes lack of a discernible cause or trigger – are the physical symptoms that accompany such intense emotions. It varies depending on the individual, but a person can suffer from headaches, muscle tension, chest pains, irregular or rapid heartbeats, insomnia, breathlessness, and other similar symptoms. Oftentimes, especially when the physical symptoms begin before the emotional roller coaster that comes with a panic attack, a person can seek medical help for the physical symptoms alone. It can often feel like one is having a heart attack, or that death is imminent because one's heartbeat has become so rapid.

The good news is that, barring any other physical condition, these physical symptoms are often simply caused by a rush of adrenaline typical of a fight or flight response, which means that one is not in any immediate danger. It is, of course, always a good idea to seek the professional opinion of your doctor to verify that these symptoms aren't caused by another physical or medical condition.

- *That the proper way to address Anxiety Disorders is by isolating yourself and avoiding social contact.*

A person who refuses to admit that there is anything wrong, and opts instead for self-isolation and avoidance of stressful social situations is already experiencing one of the many debilitating effects of Anxiety Disorders – the severe diminishing of one's ability to function well in normal and daily social situations. It might even seem logical to avoid stressful situations so that one's condition doesn't get worse, but is not a healthy option in the long run. All this does is reinforce your fear or worry, and sooner or later, another or a similar stressful situation will crop up again. And this simply cannot be helpful for a person suffering from Generalized Anxiety Disorder (GAD), for whom day-to-day things such as work, money, or relationships are the primary cause of worry. There are only so many things you can avoid for so long a time.

Without taking any proactive means of addressing one's excessive worries and fears, these symptoms can only grow worse with time. Despite a person's denials and self-imposed solitude, the undeniable reality is that one's condition has already grown to be a serious illness affecting one's ability to function well in day-to-day life. This isn't "management" but denial and avoidance.

- *That social anxiety is the same as shyness or introversion.*

In the same way that everyone can suffer from anxieties and worries without having an anxiety or a panic attack that is classified as an Anxiety Disorder, people can suffer from shyness or introversion without having the social anxiety that is classified as an Anxiety Disorder. The two are simply not the same. The key difference is in the pervasiveness and excessive impact of the physical and emotional impact that one experiences in Social Anxiety or Social Phobia that affects one's capacity to live a normal life and their ability to function well in daily life.

- *That Anxiety Disorders aren't that common.*

The truth is that Anxiety Disorders are one of the more common and prevalent psychiatric conditions in the world today. It is estimated to affect approximately 40 million adults per year in the United States alone, with one in every five adults expected to suffer from an Anxiety Disorder at some point during their lifetime.

- *That Anxiety always stems from a specific trauma or fear.*

Not always, and a specific fear or trauma certainly doesn't account for some types of Anxiety Disorders such as Generalized Anxiety Disorder (GAD) or Social Anxiety Disorder. Without having the burden of a previous trauma or a terrible experience in their past, an Anxiety Disorder can still be very real.

Of course, some types of Anxiety Disorders are particularly linked to such specific fears or traumas, for instance, specific phobias and Post-traumatic stress disorder (PTSD), but this isn't always necessarily true.

- *That Anxiety Disorders are irreversible because they are caused by chemical imbalance in the brain, a genetic predisposition, or a biological problem with the brain.*

There are myriad causes for Anxiety Disorders, and setting one's mind up to believe that they cannot be addressed effectively with therapy because they are physiological in nature only keeps one from embracing possible potential treatments that may actually be quite effective not only in managing but in effectively treating and recovering from this condition.

Even worse, it often makes people believe that because the problems are chemical or physiological in nature, that the only possible treatment is medication. But while medication does have its uses, it is unhealthy to believe that it is the only possible recourse for a person suffering from Anxiety Disorders, especially when there are behavioral therapies that can be quite effective and far more long-lasting in impact.

History of Anxiety Disorders

Anxiety and its related emotions such as worry, fear, and nervousness have always been part of the human condition, and it also has its uses as a self-preservation mechanism by helping to stimulate a person's fight or flight response to perceived threats. But the excessive fear or worry that characterizes Anxiety Disorders, in some of its earliest forms, certainly had its prejudicial and even religious overtones.

In ancient Greece, the word "hysteria" was used for women prone to anxiety. It was used primarily for women, because it was believed that such behavior derived from disturbances caused by the uterus. Female semen was also considered a culprit that needed sex to address hysterical behavior. Rather unfortunately, hysteria has since been ascribed primarily to women for the next couple of hundred years, with hysteria being seen as a sign of a witch, or later on as insanity that warranted confinement and extreme psychiatric treatments.

At the same time, other forms of Anxiety Disorder were being identified by other names. During the middle ages, for instance, and deriving from Latin *anxieties*, anxiety was much connected with Christianity's concepts of sin, confession, conscience, and the fear or worry of eternal judgment. A somewhat recognizable form of post-traumatic stress disorder was also recognized among the soldiers of the American Civil War, though it was then referred to as "irritable heart syndrome" or "nerve weakness." Also rather unfortunately, one of the prescribed treatments then was the use of opium.

Throughout the next few years, what is now termed as Anxiety Disorders have been known by other names. "Melancholy" was recognized in the 17th century based on

Robert Burton's "The Anatomy of Melancholia." Later on, after the 1800s, the French spoke of *"angoisse,"* the Germans of *"angst,"* the Spanish of *"angustia,"* and the British of *"panic."* In all these varying terminologies, care was taken to distinguish the condition from what is normal worry or fear, and instead used such heavy terminology as anguish, terror, and misery. Treatment options were of the type that, in hindsight, could only seem to add to the person's fears or worries: from electroshock therapy, fear exposure therapy, and even to sterilization to avoid passing on their "mental illness" to their children. Later on, anti-depressants were utilized as primary treatment for both anxiety and depression.

In 1980, Anxiety Disorders were recognized by the American Psychiatric Association, and since then, further widespread research has shown how severe are the disabilities caused by Anxiety Disorders – things which were initially written off as simply nerves or stress. Today, it is one of the most common mental health disorders in the world, affecting about 273 million people globally as of 2010. Thankfully, it is also one of the most treatable.

With the increase in knowledge and information on Anxiety Disorders, more and more people have been approaching medical professionals for diagnosis and treatment. And while many of the different types of Anxiety Disorders recognized today still seem to be more prevalent among women, it is unsure whether this is because of an actual greater occurrence among women, or because there are more women than men who have sought help, and thus been diagnosed with the disorder.

Chapter Two: Causes of Anxiety Disorder

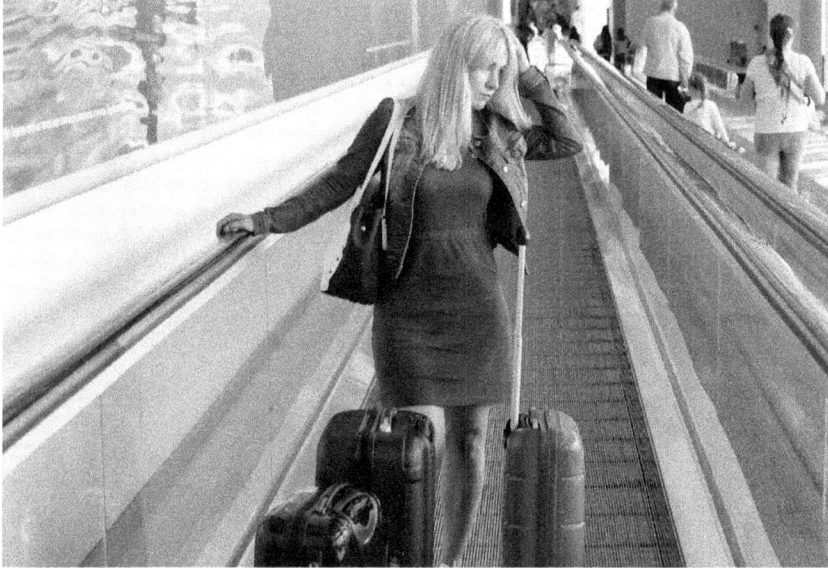

The causes of Anxiety Disorders are myriad, and far from being straight cut. If anything, this is usually caused by a combination of different factors and their unique interaction with each other that can serve to affect a person to the extent that they develop an Anxiety Disorder. Of course, each person is different, but with continued research, scientists have all but debunked the notion that Anxiety Disorders are caused by any personal weaknesses, low intelligence, poor upbringing, or individual flaws or imperfections.

In this chapter, we take a look at some of the more common causes of Anxiety Disorders, bearing in mind that it is usually a combination of two or more of the following possible causes that can effectively result in a person developing an Anxiety Disorder. There is no single factor that could single-handedly cause anxiety, which means that even if you find yourself exposed to one or more of the following possible causes, it does not necessarily mean that you will suffer from an Anxiety Disorder. This is important to remember because sometimes, anticipating or being worried about suffering from an anxiety attack can only make things worse when and if it does take place.

The following have been identified as potential causes of Anxiety Disorders, or as a crucial risk factor in the development of this condition.

Changes in Brain Function

Ascribed to being one of the potential effects of long-term exposure to stress, changes in the way our brain functions may conceivably contribute to the development of Anxiety Disorders.

Strong emotions, possible changes in the function of brain circuits, and the way nerve cells transmit information could also affect the way we process emotions such as fear and anxiety.

Environmental Stress

Significant stressful events in our immediate environment can also contribute to the possible development of Anxiety Disorders. Major life changes, illnesses, loss, or trauma, for instance, could have us reaching too deeply into our well of emotions.

Ongoing stress in our daily life that goes on for a too long period of time can also lead to chronic anxiety or panic attacks, such as a stressful job, a stressful family or home life, or the ongoing presence of some form of abuse in a person's familial or social relationship could naturally lead to some form of worry or anxiety. If the environmental causes are also ongoing, then it makes it more likely that the anxiety or panic attacks could develop into an Anxiety Disorder.

Genetics

While this has yet to be proven, and the particular genetic markers identified, Anxiety Disorders do seem to run in families, thereby arguing strongly for what could be a biological basis. What this tells us is that there could be a greater likelihood for a person having an Anxiety Disorder if someone in their family also suffers from the same condition. Traumatic or stressful events or major life changes can offer trigger this condition if one has inherited a predisposition for anxiety.

Of course, being at higher risk because of a family history of anxiety or other mental health condition does not necessarily mean that you will also experience the same thing. Genetics aside, each individual is still different, including the way they react to stress and deal with fears, worries and anxieties.

Medical Causes

Sometimes, Anxiety Disorders can easily be traced to something medical or even physiological in nature – whether a different health issue or illness altogether, or as a side-effect of medication or drugs that are being taken. This is particularly true if a person's life has not been characterized by anything excessively stressful or traumatic, there is no family history of anxiety, and you have never suffered from any bouts of anxiety before, whether during your childhood or throughout your life changes and events.

It is certainly possible that certain medications you may be taking can have the unintended side effect of anxiety or even depression. It is also possible that such emotions can be caused by another medical problem, for instance, heart disease, diabetes, respiratory problems, asthma, rare tumors, or dementia. In fact, some physical conditions can even mimic of be indistinguishable from the symptoms suffered during an anxiety attack – for instance, an overactive thyroid. On the other hand, anxiety can also take place together with other and separate mental disorders, such as depression. In this case, the more effective treatment should be targeted for both or all conditions being experienced, instead of one or the other exclusively.

This is the reason why getting a professional diagnosis is important. If the anxiety you are feeling is caused by another health condition, then the best way of treating your anxiety is by treating the underlying cause. Rule out other possible causes of the anxiety you may be feeling – this will help you to get appropriate treatment for the appropriate condition you are experiencing.

Personality Type

It seems that certain personality types are more prone to developing Anxiety Disorders than others. Shyness or inhibition during childhood seems to put some people at higher risk of developing Anxiety Disorders when they grow older. This is also true for children who lack self-esteem, are controlling or perfectionists, and are timid or inhibited. Such personality traits sometimes seem to make it more likely that a person will suffer from an anxiety attack at some point in their lives.

Drugs or alcohol

Some people do turn to drugs or alcohol to "take the edge off" when suffering from frequent anxiety attacks. One of the more common but inappropriate advice that a person with Anxiety Disorder may hear is to "have a drink or two" to settle one's nerves. The truth is that while some temporary relief might be derived from either alcohol or drugs, turning to these for "treatment" will only aggravate one's condition in the long run. Once their effects wear off, the anxiety is still there, and perhaps stronger than ever. In addition, a person may end up developing a problem with either substance abuse or alcohol abuse. And in trying to get back on track, the withdrawal symptoms that a person may experience in trying to recover from these addictive substances can certainly cause excessive anxiety.

In addition to substance and alcohol abuse, other possible causes or factors that could cause or worsen anxiety disorders are the taking of caffeine, benzodiazepine dependence, or even chronic exposure to some form of organic solvents in the environment. Actually, even moderate use of alcohol, if prolonged over a certain period of time, could contribute to the increase of anxiety attacks in certain individuals.

Chapter Three: Symptoms and Diagnosis of Anxiety Disorders

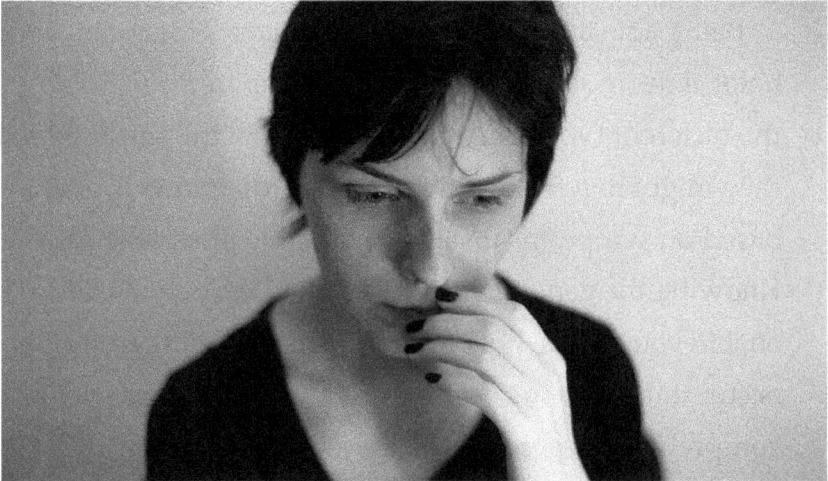

There are different types of Anxiety Disorders, and the symptoms and causes might differ depending on which type you suffer from. But there are general signs we can look to that can constitute warning signs of when you might be suffering from an anxiety attack.

Even if you have been diagnosed with a particular type of Anxiety Disorder, for instance, knowing what are considered common symptoms can be helpful because many people can suffer from more than one type at the same time. So while you may not be experiencing symptoms you have

already associated with the Anxiety Disorder type you have
been diagnosed with, you will still be able to identify the
onset of an anxiety attack, albeit of a different type.

Being able to identify the relevant symptoms can also be
helpful during diagnosis. Due to the extreme variability in
the different types of Anxiety Disorders, the age at which
they might manifest, and the degree, diagnosis is often
based on symptoms instead of tangible physiological signs.
Knowing the general symptoms of an Anxiety Disorder will
enable you to take note of them when and if they should
occur, thus enabling you to provide your doctor with a
comprehensive personal history.

For that matter, knowing the symptoms of an anxiety
disorder can help you distinguish whether what you are
experiencing is simply normal anxiety that any person can
likely expect during the course of his or her life, or whether
your experience can already be classified as an Anxiety
Disorder. Of course, a proper diagnosis should still be made
by a medical professional. A section on diagnosis of Anxiety
Disorders is provided later on in this chapter.

Symptoms of Anxiety Disorder

The symptoms of an Anxiety Disorder can range from extreme or intense emotions, physical symptoms, or certain character behaviors. Below we present you with a checklist of the signs and symptoms of an Anxiety Disorder, grouped according to these three experiential levels.

Emotional Signs and Symptoms

- Irrational and crippling fear
- Excessive worrying
- Persistent self-doubt
- An intolerance of uncertainty
- Feelings of panic, fear and uneasiness

Physical Signs and Symptoms

- Insomnia or other forms of sleep problems, and sleep disorders such as frequent nightmares, restless leg syndrome, and bruxism (gnashing of teeth during sleep)

- Chronic pain, persistent and pervasive muscle
  tension, chest pains
- Gastrointestinal disorders, digestive problems,
  frequent urination, and Irritable Bowel Syndrome
  (IBS)
- Heart Disease or other forms of heart problems
  such as racing heartbeat and heart palpitations
- Respiratory problems and shortness of breath
- Allergic reactions
- Nausea and vomiting
- Chills, twitching, shaking, and hot flashes
- Dry mouth
- Dizziness and fainting spells
- Numbness or tingling in the hands and feet

Behavioral or Medical Signs and Symptoms

- Repeated panic attacks that are characterized by
  sudden and intense fear and helplessness, coupled
  with a racing heartbeat, sweating, dizziness,
  stomach pain, and breathing problems

- Extreme stage fright and self-consciousness in social situations as possible symptoms of Social Anxiety Disorder
- Sudden flashbacks to a traumatic memory or event in the past
- Extreme and debilitating perfectionism
- Rituals that are comprised of obsessive thoughts and compulsive behavior
- Restlessness and the inability to be still and calm

In addition to the signs and symptoms enumerated above, there are certain lifestyle and environmental factors that can also contribute to a person having an Anxiety Disorder. If you have experienced or are going through any of the following, there is a greater risk that what you are experiencing may already be classified as an Anxiety Disorder:

Contributory Factors:

- Substance and alcohol abuse
- Side effects of certain drugs such as those for high blood pressure, diabetes, and thyroid disorders

- Withdrawal symptoms due to cessation of drugs, alcohol, or any medication prescribed for anxiety and sleep disorders
- Exposure to persistent and ongoing stressful environmental factors at work, school, or at home, or a specific triggering event characterized by high stress

Diagnosing Anxiety Disorders

Fear and anxiety are an important part of the human emotional repertoire – these, along with the accompanying burst of energy that comes during high stress situations, enable people to react quickly and appropriately to threats or danger, and also enables them to strive for challenging goals. It is when such emotional and physical states are disproportionate to environmental situations, excessive, prolonged, or unexpected, that it becomes irrational and paralyzing. With no external threat perceived, for instance, the energy has nowhere to go, and all that we have is a person suffering from what feels more like an anxiety or a panic attack.

But even anxiety or panic attacks do not automatically constitute an Anxiety Disorder. Most individuals are estimated to suffer from some form of anxiety or panic attack at some point in their lives. Even if the anxiety or panic you are feeling seems excessive, it might have been brought on by other factors such as a stressful life change, excessive caffeine use, lack of sleep, or other contributory factors. Again, this does not automatically mean that you have an Anxiety Disorder.

Diagnosis of Anxiety Disorders should be conducted by a medical professional. But because there is no specific causative agent or biological marker that has been identified as a sure sign of an Anxiety Disorder, a diagnosis for Anxiety Disorder is clinical rather than laboratory, and based on findings resulting from one or more of the following:

- A complete physical examination, including blood, urine or other tests that could rule out other possible medical conditions
- Complete personal and family medical history
- Interviews and diagnostic tests such as self-assessment questionnaires

These findings are used to rule out other possible causes of the signs and symptoms you are experiencing, because there are other medical conditions that yield the same symptoms as an Anxiety Disorder. Being able to thus identify which is the actual cause for your symptoms can help in identifying the most appropriate treatment methods.

Some of the possible medical conditions that your doctor should rule out before arriving at a diagnosis of Anxiety Disorder include:

- Heart Problems including a heart attack or a mitral valve prolapse
- Asthma
- Hyperthyroidism
- Hypoglycemia (low blood sugar)
- Recurrent pulmonary emboli
- Adrenal gland tumors
- Angina
- Tachycardia
- Menopause

Needless to say, other contributory factors should also be ruled out, so it is advisable for you to be completely honest with your doctor about any possible history you may have in using alcohol, drugs, medication, or specific stressful events or situations you may have experienced, or are experiencing.

Once other possible medical conditions are ruled out, your doctor will then refer you to a psychiatrist, psychologist or other mental health professional specializing in the diagnosis and treatment of mental illnesses. They will continue your examination using interviews and various assessment tools, including an evaluation of the severity, degree, and intensity of the symptoms you are experiencing, including their own observation of your behavior and attitude. All these enable them to identify whether you are in fact suffering from an Anxiety Disorder, and which type.

In general, however, and based on the overall results of your evaluation, it is when the symptoms you are feeling have been present for at least six months, are disproportional to your situation, and have effectively diminished your ability to function normally, then it is a very likely that you are suffering from some form of Anxiety Disorder. The actual diagnosis is mainly based on differential diagnostic criteria which differs for each type of Anxiety Disorder.

Chapter Three: Symptoms and Diagnosis of Anxiety Disorders

Chapter Four: Types of Anxiety Disorders

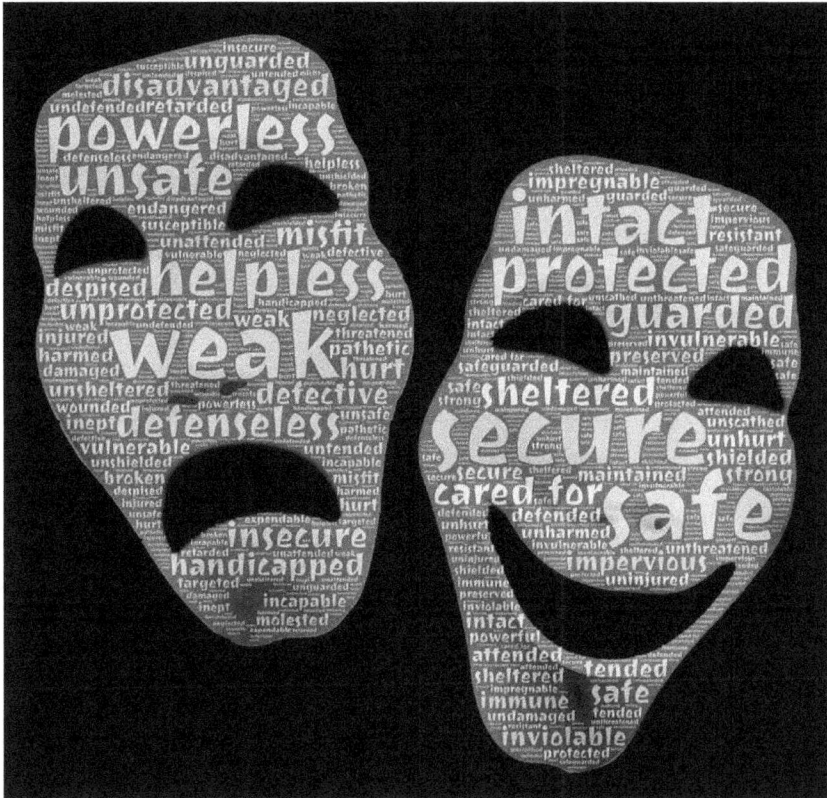

There are over 60 different conditions or diseases that are considered as subtypes of dementia, and several ways of classifying or categorizing them. In this chapter, we look at some of these major classifications, and also at some of the more common subtypes or causes of dementia.

Different Types of Anxiety Disorders

Generalized Anxiety Disorder (GAD)

Symptoms: excessive and irratonal worry about everyday matters, fatigue, headaches, nausea, muscle tension, diarrhea, difficulty breathing, insomnia, restlessness, irritability

Possible Causes: Genetics or family history, substance use, stressful life events, psychological factors and certain personality traits

Recommended Treatment: Cognitive Behavioral Therapy (CBT) and medication

Comorbidities: Depression, substance abuse, irritable bowel syndrome, insomnia, headaches, ADHD

Outlook: The symptoms are expected to still recur from time to time, and there is no "cure" that would remove the GAD completely, but the symptoms can be managed, and substantial relief afforded the individual

Generalized Anxiety Disorder is so named because there is usually little to no specific reason for worry, other than a generalized worry or anxiety over everyday things such as health, responsibilities, money, repairs, keeping appointments, etc. There is trouble controlling such constant worries, and a person may often be unable to relax and is usually easily startled. There may also be physical symptoms accompanying the constant worrying such as fatigue, muscle tension, and a difficulty sleeping and concentrating, irritability, twitching or sweating, and a difficulty swallowing.

A person who often worries about everything about daily life may also have difficulty making decisions and remembering commitments, because what is foremost in their minds are the worries and the anticipation of disaster or possible negative events and consequences, even when there is little reason to worry or there is no apparent reason for concern.

This is considered one of the most prevalent type of Anxiety Disorders, and affects some 6.8 million adults in the United States alone, and about 4% of people worldwide, being more common among women than men.

GAD transpires gradually, and while a person with GAD may still be able to function normally, certain severe episodes of anxiety such as times of stress may cause difficulties even in simple daily routines and activities. The difficulty, of course, is that what should be considered the normal ups and downs of daily life are, in themselves, the reason for the excessive and unwarranted emotional rollercoaster of dread, fear, nervousness and worry.

Panic Disorder

Symptoms: sudden and unpredictable recurrent panic attacks characterized by intense fear, heart palpitations, shaking, shortness of breath, sweating, and a feeling of something terrible about to happen

Possible Causes: Genetics or family history, smoking, traumatic history, stress, alcohol, excessive use of stimulants and/or sedatives

Recommended Treatment: Counseling, CBT, and medication

Comorbidities: Clinical depression, personality disorders, specific phobias, Generalized Anxiety Disorder, Post-traumatic Stress Disorder, Agoraphobia

Outlook: with proper treatment, prognosis is generally good, with a high chance (90%) of finding relief

Panic Disorder occurs when a person suffers from recurring episodes of panic attacks. A panic attack is characterized by intense fear or terror that is also accompanied by physical manifestations such as shaking, sweating, dizziness, faintness, chest pains, palpitations, and a shortness of breath. Many people suffer from panic attacks at some point in their lives, but if such panic attacks are both recurrent and disabling and has been taking place for more than a month, a person may be suffering from a panic disorder.

The rush of physical, mental and emotional sensations experienced during a panic attack is far more severe and intense when compared to those experienced in a GAD, and these can last from several minutes to longer, usually peaking at 10 minutes, and never lasting for more than an hour. Sometimes, mental distress can even be suffered at the fear of getting another panic attack. This is because panic attacks can be experienced without any noticeable trigger and just seemingly comes out of nowhere – it can sometimes happen even during sleep. The unpredictability of when it might happen again can make people anxious and worried about when it might next strike.

The range of physical and emotional sensations can all be experienced in a matter of minutes, and all the while a person undergoes a terrible feeling of impending doom or the feeling that they are about to die, and a concomitant feeling of helplessness. Needless to say, if left undiagnosed and untreated, a person with panic disorder can find a severe deterioration in the quality of life that he or she can lead.

The physical symptoms can often be so tangible and debilitating that a person experiencing a series of panic attacks will seek medical attention for these physical symptoms alone, fearing that something may be physically wrong with them. The truth is that a person may sometimes experience a panic attack with the physical symptoms taking place before the actual feeling of anxiety or fear, so the worry about physical health is often justified. In any case, seeking professional medical help is always advisable in order for the panic disorder to be properly diagnosed and treated.

Agoraphobia

Symptoms: fear of certain situations or places, need to escape, severe anxiety, fear of losing control, and panic attacks with physical symptoms such as racing heartbeat, shortness of breath, trembling, dizziness, choking, and nausea

Possible Causes: Genetics or family history, other similar phobias such as claustrophobia and social phobia, depression, substance abuse, other anxiety disorders such as GAD or OCD, previous trauma such as bereavement or a history of abuse, previous incidence of a panic attack, difficulties with spatial orientation

Recommended Treatment: therapy such as Cognitive Behavior Therapy and Exposure Therapy, and medication

Comorbidities: Panic attacks. Separation anxiety disorder

Outlook: this is a lifelong disorder that requires ongoing treatment, but early intervention and treatment can help in managing the symptoms, and the levels or degrees of progress that a person can make can be very substantial. If Agoraphobia persists without any treatment or intervention, it may progressively worsen and become harder to treat

Agoraphobia is a fear of places and situations that a person perceives as dangerous or uncomfortable. When a person finds himself or herself in an undesirable situation or a feared place, they can feel helpless, scared, trapped, or panicked. Many of the other symptoms of a panic attack can also take place, including nausea and a rapid heartbeat.

Usually diagnosed during early adulthood, this can be a debilitating condition because the stress that a person experiences can be so severe that they end up avoiding doing anything else, and far prefers to stay isolated in their homes the rest of the day, thus interfering with the normal day to day activities, including their job or school performance and their personal relationships.

The accompanying panic attacks can be so frightening that a person ends up avoiding everyday places for fear of once again suffering another attack. Because the average onset of this condition is around 20 years of age, a person can end up fearing or avoiding places and situations he or she once enjoyed, such as crowded malls, supermarkets, church, theaters, etc. In fact, the term originally derives from Greek, which literally translates to "fear of the marketplace." In a very real sense, however, it isn't precisely fear of a certain place (though certain places might grow to have certain fearful associations), but fear of suffering attacks in certain places, and of suffering the concomitant frustration, worry, social embarrassment, and shame of losing control in those places – for instance, in crowded places, public transportation, roads or highways while driving, etc. On the other hand, some instances of Agoraphobia are less a fear of crowded places and more a fear of being alone and isolated.

The very real danger for a person suffering from Agoraphobia is that the resulting avoidance of certain places and locations can lead to the unintentional creation of "safety zones" or "comfort areas" where one believes that he or she is safe and protected. This can lead to self-isolation and unhealthy avoidance issues and behavior. Exposure therapy under the guidance of a qualified medical professional is therefore one of the recommended methods of treatment.

It is estimated by the National Institute of Mental Health (NIMH) that some 0.8 percent of adults suffer from agoraphobia, and 40% of such cases are considered severe.

Social Anxiety Disorder

Symptoms: self-consciousness, fear of being judged negatively, blushing, dry mouth, excessive sweating, stammering, muscle twitches, trembling, difficulty swallowing, shortness of breath, upset stomach, feelings of inadequacy, inferiority, embarrassment, humiliation, and depression

Possible Causes: May run in families, environmental atmosphere in the family where a person has underdeveloped social skills, is often being criticized, or when a parent is overprotective and exaggerates the dangers of speaking to strangers

Recommended Treatment: therapy such as Cognitive Behavior Therapy or Talk Therapy, medication

Comorbidities: Body Dysmorphic Order (BDD) or body-image anxiety disorder, panic attacks, depression, generalized anxiety disorder, post-traumatic stress disorder

Outlook: can become chronic and pervasive, but with proper treatment, this condition can be overcome.

In brief, Social Anxiety Disorder is the fear of interacting with and being judged by other people, but to a degree that is far more excessive than simple introversion. Everyone has moments of embarrassment, shyness, self-consciousness, or fear of some form of confrontation or interaction with another person, but when the fear becomes so intense that you begin avoiding all possible triggers (which is essentially most or all social interactions), thus disrupting the normal course of your life, it becomes a disorder.

Previously referred to as "social phobia," there are two types of social anxiety disorder. The more specific type is fear of specific situations such as having stage fright or fear of speaking in public. A more generalized type of social anxiety disorder is a fear or anxiety around being involved in almost all types of social situations – whether it is meeting someone new, being the center of attention, being watched by other people, speaking on the phone, meeting authority figures, and other similar social situations. Needless to say, social relationships, whether of friendship, familial, work related, or even romantic, tends to suffer for people with this disorder. This is especially true when you begin to feel the need to always have a friend accompany you wherever you go.

The frustration that people with Social Anxiety Disorder suffer from the most is that while they may be perceived as aloof, withdrawn, unfriendly or uninterested, they are actually oftentimes desirous of forming social relationships and being included. The difficulty is that they are held back by extreme low self-esteem, and a fear of being criticized or judged negatively. Even though they may recognize that their fears are irrational, they are often powerless against the extreme anxiety that they experience. Unfortunately, rather than seeking professional help, some people who suffer from Social Anxiety Disorder "self-medicate" by using drugs or alcohol. Needless to say, doing so will only worsen the condition, and likely lead to other problems such as alcoholism, substance abuse, eating disorders, etc.

This is considered to be the third largest psychological disorder in the country, and it is estimated that millions of people globally suffer from this condition.

Specific Phobias

Symptoms: trembling, dizziness, sweating, racing heartbeat, extreme and uncontrollable fear, choking, nausea, faintness, chest pains, going out of your way to avoid feared objects or situations

Possible Causes: May run in families, particularly within the first degree, temperament, a previous traumatic event, loss or abuse, overprotectiveness of parents, learned reactions to specific objects or situations

Recommended Treatment: therapy such as targeted psychotherapy or cognitive behavioral therapy; medication is generally not recommended unless in certain severe situations

Comorbidities: panic attacks

Outlook: specific phobias are treatable through psychological treatments and therapy, sometimes in combination with medication

As its name implies, this is a condition where a person has an excessive, persistent, and uncontrollable fear or phobia of a specific object or situation, even though it poses no immediate or actual danger or threat. The anxiety reaction is out of proportion or exaggerated in relation to the cause of the fear. While there is a recognition that the fear itself is often irrational and unwarranted, the feeling of fear that arises when met by the situation is, in itself, uncontrollable.

The beginnings of specific phobias can often be traced to childhood or adolescence, and persists well into adulthood, but it can certainly occur at any age. While children do suffer from common fears, they eventually learn to manage their fears as they grow up. But phobias are of a different class altogether,

Individuals with specific phobias generally do not suffer from anxiety in general, but they do suffer extreme fear when confronted by a specific thing or situation – some of the more common specific phobias are fear animals (spiders or snakes), of a specific environment such (e.g., water or heights), blood, a specific situation such as flying, tunnels, enclosed spaces, or other phobia types such as a fear of clowns, loud sounds, fear of choking, etc. There are some individuals that can actually suffer from multiple phobias.

When the thing or situation that is feared is rare enough, people may not find it necessary to seek help. It is when the thing or object is expected to transpire in daily life, and a person anticipates the feared object or situation so much that he or she avoids it, or suffers a panic attack, thus disrupting the normal course of their life, that the condition becomes classified as an Anxiety Disorder. Should the individual have no choice but to go through the feared experience, they will do so under great distress. For children, their fear or dread of the thing or situation that is feared can often manifest as tantrums, crying, clinging, or freezing.

Oftentimes, a person can make life decisions based on whether or not they will come into contact with their phobias, thus limiting many of their opportunities. When actually faced with the thing, object or situation feared, a person can suffer from a severe panic attack.

Separation Anxiety Disorder

Symptoms: extreme distress at being separated from certain people or from home, persistent worry or fear at possible harm or danger befalling oneself or the figure to whom one is attached, avoidance of activities that might result in separation, repeated nightmares, refusal to go to school, refusal to sleep alone, fear of being alone, physical complaints such as headaches, nausea, stomachaches, general aches and pains, shortness of breath, sweating, or vomiting, feelings of helplessness, anger, sadness, shame, worry and fear

Possible Causes: May run in families, or environmental, such as a general feeling of lack of safety that might be caused by environmental changes, stress, or having been raised in an overprotective environment; if it seems to transpire overnight, it might be caused by a traumatic experience such as the loss of a loved one, death or divorce

Recommended Treatment: therapy such as cognitive behavior treatment, talk therapy, play therapy, or counseling; and exercises such as relaxation, coping strategies, role-playing, and reinforcement; medication may sometimes be used in severe cases

Comorbidities: depression, dysthymic disorder, major depressive disorder, generalized anxiety disorder, may sometimes be followed by panic disorder and agoraphobia, specific phobias, PTSD, panic disorder, obsessive-compulsive disorders

Outlook: prognosis is good, this disorder is very treatable especially when caught early and appropriate treatment is given, although the symptoms may recur for many years, especially during stressful situations or events.

Separation Anxiety Disorder happens when a person experiences excessive or intense anxiety at the thought of separation from a person to whom one is attached. It occurs most often in children between 8-14 months who grew up among close-knit families when they experience separation from major attachment figures in their family or from home, but this disorder can also occur among adolescents and adults.

While many children do suffer some discomfort at being separated from people or situations we feel safe with, the anxiety suffered in Separation Anxiety Disorder is persistent and excessive beyond what can normally be expected. When despite reassurances and the best efforts of parents, the separation anxiety experienced by the child persists for a long time and becomes disruptive, it is considered a disorder.

When separation does occur, a person becomes withdrawn, sad, apathetic, or has difficulty concentrating on work or at play. Anger may be displayed towards the person enforcing the separation. Some may also suffer from fears of dangerous situations that may transpire while they are alone, such as accidents, burglars, monsters, etc., or of harm befalling the person to whom they are attached. A more severe result is that a person (particularly children) might end up feeling that they are unloved or have been abandoned.

Such personalities that suffer from Separation Anxiety Disorder can have difficult social relationships because others perceive them as attention-seeking, demanding, and clingy. Needless to say, the anxiety felt and behavior displayed due to the separation, and the demanding personality exhibited by such individuals make it difficult to have a normal daily routine, thus having a disruptive effect in their lives and social development.

Obsessive-compulsive disorder (OCD)

Symptoms: obsessive thoughts, compulsions, routines or rituals, a fear that things not being done a certain way might cause some potential tragedy, emotions such as anger, shame or guilt, and physical symptoms such as stomachaches, headaches, muscle tension, shortness of breath, and a racing heartbeat

Possible Causes: not precisely known, but is suspected to be the result of a combination of biological and environmental factors, including abnormalities in certain areas of the brain, traumatic life events and certain personality types also seem to be contributory factors

Recommended Treatment: counselling, support groups, and therapy such as cognitive behavioral therapy and psychotherapy; medication may often be prescribed to relieve symptoms, but not in effecting lasting treatment

Comorbidities: Body Dysmorphic Disorder (BDD), Compulsive skin picking (CSP), Trichotillomania (urge to pull out one's hair), hoarding compulsion, Obsessive-compulsive personality disorder, Tic Disorder

Outlook: the condition is treatable with professional guidance and a supportive network

Commonly known as OCD, Obsessive-compulsive Disorder is characterized by obsessions and repetitive or intrusive thoughts, and the need to ease one's anxieties by the performance of ritualistic behaviors and routines or compulsions that one feels compelled to perform.

Obsessive thoughts are often repetitive, disturbing and distracting, while compulsions are rituals or behaviors that one feels the need to repeat over and over again. Such constant, senseless repetition are often irrational and serve no purpose whatsoever, and as such ultimately end up being intrusive and disrupting, not to mention time-consuming. What relief that acting on these obsessions and compulsions may give a person with their anxiety or distress is inevitably temporary. Anxiety recurs, possibly stronger than ever, and the OCD symptoms become recurring and loops around like a broken record or CD.

Even though such obsessions and compulsions often grow to become intrusive to a person's normal routine, a person with OCD simply cannot help but engage in such senseless and pointless routines in order to ward off persistent and unwelcome thoughts or feelings. Some of these obsessions or compulsions include the need to double-check things repeatedly, frequent hand-washes with an irrational fear of germs; perfectionists with a need to double check everything usually act under the impression that something terrible will happen if they make a mistake, hoarders with an irrational fear of throwing anything away, or those obsessed with symmetry and order who continually count and arrange things in their environment to bring things in line with certain inner criteria. Some obsessive thoughts center around religious ideals, superstitions, and a fear of losing control.

If OCD goes untreated, it can severely hamper a person's life. While people usually have mild forms of OCD symptoms, these are often manageable. It is when the symptoms are so severe that they interfere with work or school, relationships, and even one's capacity to live a fruitful life that it becomes an Anxiety Disorder. This is because most of a person's time and energy is being consumed by these obsessions and compulsions.

Perhaps one of the greatest frustrations that a person with OCD may experience is how the condition is perceived by other people. Many people see it as nothing more than a desire to keep repeating something over and over again, not so different from what everybody else goes through during certain times in their life, and nothing more. In reality, it is extremely disruptive to a person's life, and the anxiety and distress that it causes is also very real.

Post-traumatic Stress Disorder (PTSD)

Symptoms: flashbacks or nightmares that remind you of a traumatic event, physical reactions to memories of those events such as sweating, nausea, etc., extreme avoidance of reminders of the trauma, emotional numbness, irritability, difficulty concentrating, hypervigilance or constantly being "on alert," shame or guilt, depression, distrust, aggression, work or relationship problems

Possible Causes: triggered by traumatic or threatening events, past history of trauma, previous mental health problems, ongoing stressful live events after the trauma, absence of social support

Recommended Treatment: counseling, therapy such as cognitive behavioral therapy, talk therapy, or Eye Movement Desensitization and Reprocessing (EMDR) therapy, medication for severe symptoms, physical activity such as exercise, calming exercises

Comorbidities: depression, specific phobias, severe anxiety, dissociative disorder, suicidal feelings

Outlook: highly variable; a person may be able to move on past the traumatic event, and others may simply learn how to cope better with the symptoms and managing to live a better quality of life

This condition has been called by many names over the years, particularly in reference to the experiences of war veterans: shell shock, soldier's heart, battle fatigue, or combat stress. Essentially, PTSD or Post-traumatic Stress Disorder is the inability to move past a traumatic event. This is usually triggered by traumatic events that threatened a person's safety or affected a person powerfully, such as disasters, war, accidents, rape or some form of abuse, kidnapping, etc. People who experience PTSD aren't limited to the victims of such events, or those who personally experience them. Sometimes, witnesses, or emergency workers that work to help people directly after such events can also suffer from PTSD

When a threatening of traumatic event takes place, you either freeze or feel immobilized, or your fight or flight response takes hold, stimulating your nervous system. Once the danger is past, the body eventually returns to normal, even if it takes some time for us to be able to move on. But for a person suffering from PTSD, things don't quite return to normal, and a person is stuck feeling upset and vulnerable, constantly bombarded with painful or terrifying memories.

When children suffer from PTSD, the symptoms they experience differ from what adults experience – for instance: bed wetting, acting out the traumatic event during play, being unusually clingy, or the development of destructive or disruptive behaviors.

Anybody can suffer from PTSD, but those whose experiences are particularly intense, if they went on for some period of time such as living in a war zone or repeated physical or sexual abuse, or those who suffered some form of injury because of such events, seem more likely to suffer from this condition. PTSD also seems more prevalent after certain events – it is most commonly associated among war veterans, and those who have suffered from rape or sexual assault.

PTSD symptoms can come and go for months or years after the triggering event. It isn't clear why some individuals are more prone to suffering from PTSD than others, but it may be due to the intensity or severity of the situation, some previous form of mental condition, or a total lack of any support system after the event. If it begins to affect a person's ability to live a normal life, then it is considered PTSD that is classified as an Anxiety Disorder.

Selective Mutism

Symptoms: speaking normally in certain settings, but is selectively mute around strange settings or around strangers, looks visibly uncomfortable or even angry when asked to speak, communicates through gestures or facial expressions instead of normal speech, appears nervous, awkward, rude, clingy, stiff, or tense, may sometimes display temper tantrums

Possible Causes: possible genetic influences and a family history of anxiety disorders, speech or language problems, the need to learn a second language

Recommended Treatment: therapy such as shaping, spacing, self-modeling, stimulus facing, desensitization, and medication

Comorbidities: severe anxiety, shyness, social anxiety, social phobia, social avoidance, depression, sensory integration dysfunction

Outlook: diagnosed early and given proper treatment, a child can successfully overcome this condition; adolescents and adults can also overcome Selective Mutism, but it becomes progressively more difficult to do so as a person matures

Selective Mutism occurs when a person who does not otherwise suffer from any speech impediment or other related conditions such as Autism does not speak to select individuals, select settings, or outside the home, but otherwise speaks and converses normally in other situations.

When confronted with the need or expectation to speak in such situations, the child freezes and experiences a feeling of panic. Talking literally becomes impossible. Eventually, they learn to avoid such situations or develop avoidant behavior.

This condition is more common among children and occurs from the ages of 1-3 years old, though it does not usually become noticeable until the ages of 3-7, or during school years when the child is expected to interact in social settings outside the home. Should it persist until adolescence, Selective Mutism becomes progressively more difficult to treat. If the condition is left untreated until adulthood, while treatment may still be possible, it could mean years of wasted opportunities for social interaction and personal growth.

The difficulty is that because most children do suffer from some form of shyness, it is assumed that the child will eventually grow out of it. At other times, it is assumed, mistakenly, that a child is simply being stubborn, or that his behavior is the result of a possible trauma. In cases of Selective Mutism, however, instead of the condition being temporary, it only worsens over time. And instead of being the result of trauma or stubbornness, there is often no prior history of trauma, and the child's mutism is more often the result of extreme inhibition rather than stubbornness. What motivates a child to display behaviors of Selective Mutism is, on the other hand, avoidant behavior that may be the result of some form of social anxiety and an irrational fear of speaking to or interacting with strangers outside of the home.

This condition causes significant impairment in the quality of a child's life, interfering with school, their ability to make friends, to expand their experiences, and to grow outside of the home setting. They may experience urinary infections because they are unable to ask to go to the bathroom, and their schoolwork may suffer because they are afraid to ask questions and seek clarification.

When this happens for an extended period of time, the condition is properly an Anxiety Disorder.

Proper diagnosis and immediate treatment and intervention is, therefore, advisable. It is important to rule out other possible causes such as speech or language delays, autism, or even anxiety that results from actual trauma. Being able to identify the correct condition allows for a proper implementation of treatment and coping strategies, where the root cause is some form of anxiety.

Chapter Five: Social Anxiety in Children

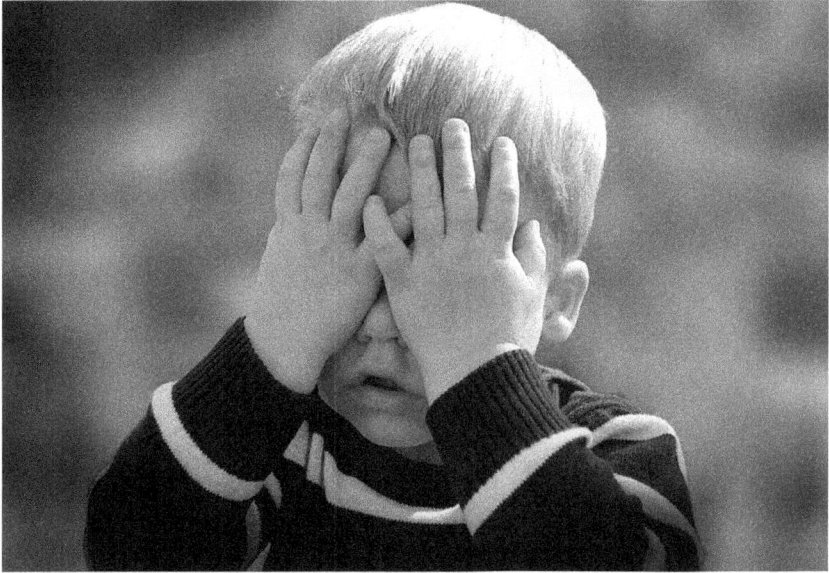

It is estimated that some 10-20 percent of children develop some form of anxiety disorder before the age of 18. Indeed, many children and adolescents suffer from some form of anxiety during certain novel experiences, and most of the time, this is a normal part of growing up.

However, sometimes children are not able to move past their anxieties, and they get stuck. Unable to expand their experiences and grow as most children are expected to, and at such a crucial time in their lives, it becomes imperative that cases of Anxiety Disorders in children are diagnosed early so that immediate and appropriate treatment may be given.

While diagnosis for each specific type of Anxiety Disorder is different, in general, the following constitute warning signs that parents and caregivers should watch out for in children:

- Worries or anxieties that cannot be helped
- The fear or worry is irrational and illogical – both to the child as well as to his or her parents
- The fear or worry does not diminish even after reassurances or explanations
- The fear or worry is so severe that it interferers with a child's normal growth and daily routines, severely hampering their ability to live a normal life

What Anxiety Disorders can a child suffer from?

Some of the types of Anxiety Disorders provided in the previous chapter could conceivably account for a child's behavior. These can include any of the following:

- Generalized Anxiety Disorder (GAD)
- Panic Disorder
- Specific Phobias
- Selective Mutism

- Social Phobia
- Separation Anxiety Disorder
- Obsessive-compulsive Disorder
- Post-traumatic Stress Disorder (PTSD)

The main difficulty, of course, is that a child's worries or fears are often seen as simply a normal part of their growing up, and parents do not often realize the extent of the problem until some considerable time afterwards.   It is estimated that some 80% of children with a diagnosable Anxiety Disorder are not getting treatment, according to the 2015 Child Mind Institute Children's Mental Health Report. This disorder affects at least one in eight children, and, when left untreated, translates to poor school performance, limited social growth and experiences, and are more likely to later on engage in substance abuse.

Be observant of your child, and pay attention should any of the following symptoms become manifest, particularly when physical and emotional symptoms begin to show without any discernible cause or reason.

- Difficulty concentrating
- Nightmares, inability to sleep alone
- Anger or irritability, throwing tantrums
- Constant worries and negative thoughts
- Not eating properly

- A constant need to use the toilet
- Being clingy and overly dependent
- Complaints of stomach aches and generally not feeling well
- Constantly crying

Tips for Parents and Caregivers of Children with Anxiety Disorders

It helps to remember that the development of Anxiety Disorders in children is not a sign of poor parenting – to this day, the precise cause or causes of Anxiety Disorders are not known, though it is theorized that it may be due to a combination of genetic and environmental factors. The important thing is not to get stuck on why the condition developed in the first place, and to focus instead on providing the proper support system that can enable your child to move past or recover from his or her anxieties.

If you have a child diagnosed with an Anxiety Disorder, or if you suspect that your child may be suffering from anxieties and worries that are out of proportion to what should be normally expected in children, here are a few tips to help you as you assist your child in managing his condition:

- Be observant; pay attention to your child's behaviors, particularly during stressful events like attending social gatherings, being around strange people and strange surroundings, or going to school for the first time, etc. This will enable you to recognize the symptoms early on, and perhaps the specific causes or triggers.
- Should your child become anxious or fearful during specific events, stay calm yourself and reassure them in a calm, soothing voice
- Praise them for accomplishments, no matter how small, but don't punish them for making mistakes or for their lack of or slow progress. Praising them for their accomplishments can help build their self-esteem and personal strength.
- Try to maintain a normal routine, but be as flexible as possible.
- Adjust your expectations, particularly during stressful periods or transitions
- Encourage independence by letting them learn things on their own, and making mistakes for which they are not punished. Try not to be over-protective, especially about everyday things such

as being alone or talking to people outside of the family.

- Should your child suffer or be exposed to traumatic or stressful experiences, provide them with a support system, and encourage self-expression as much as possible.

- Beware of your own fears and anxieties. In some instances, a child's anxieties are learned – if they see that you are fearful or anxious about something, they are likely to believe that it is something to be fearful or anxious about, as well.

- Try to include some form of positive activities and humor into your child's daily routine. This teaches them that life is about exploration, gaining new experiences, learning from mistakes, and moving on.

Chapter Six: Treatment of Anxiety Disorders

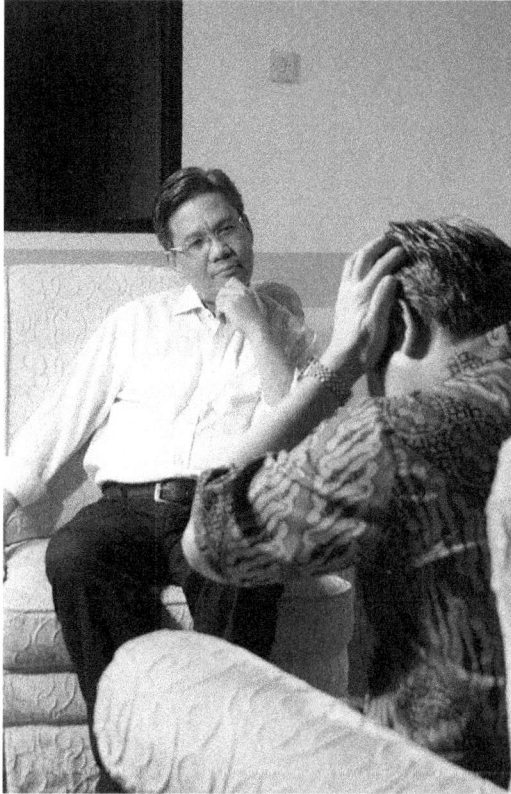

There are two main types of treatment preferred for Anxiety Disorders, and these have shown effective either separately or together. Depending on the type of Anxiety Disorder you have, the symptoms you experience, and your unique personal and medical history, the variations of type within these two main treatment types can also vary. Your primary care physician will be in the best position to prescribe which type of treatment is best for you. They should discuss your treatment options with you, making you aware of expected results and any possible consequences before treatment proper is undertaken.

These two treatment consists of:

1. Pharmacological Treatments; and
2. Psychological Treatments

Both medication and therapy are, of course, broad in application, and may conceivably vary depending on which type of specific therapy and/or medication is deemed appropriate for your personal circumstances. In this chapter, we take a closer look at the subtypes of each of these two main types of treatment for Anxiety Disorder:

Pharmacological Treatments

There are some who advocate avoiding medication altogether and sticking solely to therapy or counseling, but most doctors prefer a combined approach. Of course, it is imperative that you don't take any medication unless prescribed by your doctor, and that you follow the prescribed dosages carefully. Each pharmacological treatment is expected to have its own possible side-effects, but these are often tolerable. On the other hand, such medications have been shown to have amazing results, particularly with the more intense or severe symptoms of Anxiety Disorder.

Medication can either address psychological or physical symptoms, depending on your unique experiences. The amount and dosage should be determined by your primary care physician, and based on your unique circumstances and the degree or severity of the symptoms you suffer from. Some, for instance, only need to use them for temporary relief during moments of great stress or anxiety, while others may need to take them their entire life. Please don't forget to discuss with your doctor what the possible side-effects are, how they may interact with other medication you may be currently taking, and how long you are expected to take them. Should medication be prescribed, your progress should be periodically assessed in order to determine any adjustments that need to be made in terms of dosage. Never self-medicate, and consult with your doctor if you feel that you need to decrease your dosage, or should you suffer or experience any strange or negative side-effects.

Some of the pharmacological treatments often prescribed for persons suffering from Anxiety Disorders, and which have shown to be effective with this condition, include:

Benzodiazepines

Benzodiazepines are mostly prescribed only as needed – there is a risk of addiction in taking this drug if used for long periods of time, which means that any prescription is often set at a low and regular dose. At most, Benzodiazepines should not be used longer than four weeks at the most.

This is a type of sedative that can sometimes be used during periods of severe anxiety, and helps to temporarily ease the symptoms that a person is feeling.

Some of the side-effects that can be felt from the use of Benzodiazepines include drowsiness, vertigo, headaches, shaking or tremors, and difficult concentrating. These should not be used, therefore, when a person is expected to be alert such as when driving or operating dangerous machinery.

Selective Serotonin reuptake inhibitors (SSRIs)

This is a type of anti-depressant that works by increasing the serotonin levels in your brain.

Some of the possible side-effects that can be felt with SSRIs include diarrhea or constipation, agitation, blurred vision, dizziness, sweating, headaches, insomnia or drowsiness, sexual difficulties, and indigestion or loss of appetite

Serotonin and noradrenaline reuptake inhibitors (SNRIs)

SNRIs are another type of anti-depressant increases the amounts of both serotonin and noradrenaline in your brain, while also increasing your blood pressure.

Some of the common side-effects that you may experience with SNRIs include insomnia, headaches, drowsiness, dizziness, dry mouth, sweating, constipation, or just generally feeling sick.

Pregabalin

Pregabalin is an anti-convulsant, designed to treat seizures, but have also been found to be effective for anxiety.

Some of the side-effects of Pregabalin include dizziness, drowsiness, increased appetite, blurred, vision, vertigo, and dry mouth.

Beta-Blockers

Beta-Blockers help by giving a person relief from the physical symptoms of anxiety, such as shaking, trembling, blushing, and rapid heartbeat.

Psychological Treatments or Psychotherapy

Psychological treatments including counseling and therapy are usually the first recommendations of a doctor before medication is considered as an option. These should be suited to the unique experiences and symptoms of an individual, and generally involves talking or conversing with a professional about one's experiences regarding anxiety. The goal is to learn to manage or control your anxiety symptoms sufficiently so that they don't end up controlling you. Should a person's anxiety symptoms be so severe that professionals cannot work with them in a one-on-one setting, many psychotherapies can still be successfully carried out online or through the Internet.

Some psychological treatments that have been found to be effective for people with Anxiety Disorders include:

Cognitive Behavioral Therapy (CBT)

CBT, or Cognitive Behavioral Therapy, involves the identification of thoughts or patterns of behavior that cause anxiety, understanding and acknowledging them, and then challenging them within a safe and supported environment. Eventually, a person "learns" different ways or methods of coping with traumatic or stressful events that ultimately supplant one's anxiety response.

CBT involves slow and manageable steps that eventually help the person to overcome the causes of their fears or worries, and are conducted by a specially trained therapist.

This has often been found to be the most effective treatment method for Anxiety Disorders, but of course the results vary with each individual.

Behavior Therapy

Often provided as a component of CBT, this type of therapy involves the encouragement of positive behaviors that are intended to reverse or supplant patterns of behavior that center around worry and fear. Rather than avoidance, general exposure coupled with pleasant experiences and rewards can instead help reverse learned patterns of anxiety.

Exposure Therapy

Exposure Therapy is often conducted as a component of CBT, and involves the person engaging with the very thing that causes them fear or anxiety, while being taught various strategies or coping techniques such as relaxation exercises or visualization to help them overcome, and eventually supplant, automatic and irrational fears or anxieties.

Chapter Seven: Complementary and Alternative Treatments for Anxiety Disorders

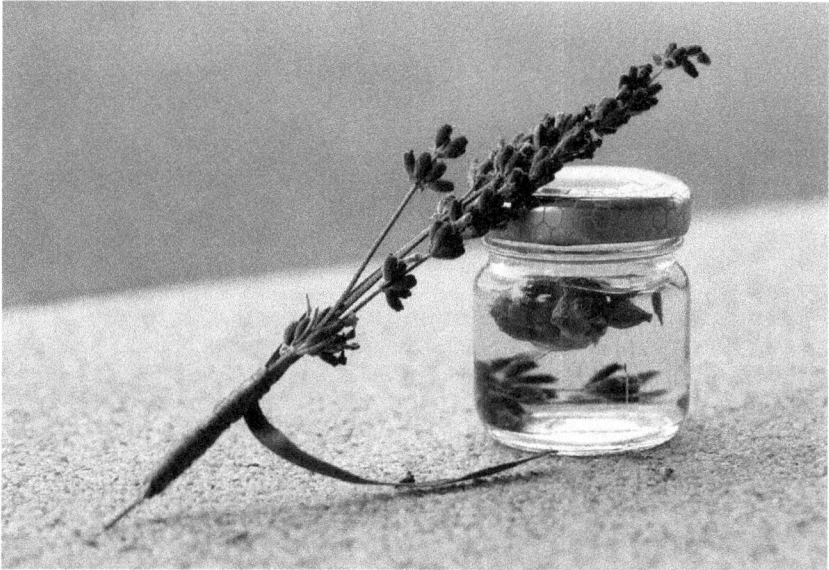

While psychotherapy and medication are the primary methods of treatment often prescribed by professionals, many doctors also seek to enhance the effects or results of treatments by prescribing complementary or alternative methods of treatment that are more holistic or natural. In general, these are not considered to be drug-based, and are not intended to be the sole focus of any treatment method. People suffering from Anxiety Disorders are still advised to focus on the main treatment types of therapy and medication.

Complementary and Alternative Treatment Methods

Relaxation Techniques

Many therapists actually include relaxation techniques into their sessions, making it an integral tool to set the mood for consultations.

Even if you aren't scheduled for any therapy, you can still explore the myriad relaxation techniques on your own. You can try meditation, yoga, tai-chi, or other forms of discipline that stress the importance of relaxation.

The ability to relax is a crucial skill, particularly for those undergoing stressful situations. The good news is that, just like any other skill, it can be learned.

Yoga, Tai Chi, and Meditation

For years, Eastern practices have been touted as exemplifying the very things that the Western world has all too often ignored.

Stillness, relaxation, taking things as they come, feeling comfortable in one's body, working with one's body, acceptance and understanding – are just some of the values that eastern practices emphasize. The lack of judgment is crucial, particularly for those suffering from Anxiety Disorders who are more likely to focus on their fears or worries of being judged, of things going wrong, or of things going out of their control. A change of mindset can help people realize that these differing mindsets are not really something to fear but to embrace.

Exercise

Even if you aren't into taking up eastern disciplines such as yoga or tai chi, even regular cardiovascular or aerobic exercise can help a great deal. Being active in some way and focusing on physical activities rather than one one's thoughts seem to help substantially for those that suffer from anxiety symptoms.

And studies seem to bear this out, as people who take up regular exercise show decreased levels of depression, and those who continue exercising even after recovery had lower risks of suffering from a relapse.

Lifestyle Changes

Most of our lifestyles in the modern world are designed to keep us on the alert in order for us to keep up with the demands of daily life. To a certain extent, being on our toes continually helps us keep up – endless workloads, the need to work harder for that next promotion, and family and social demands leaves almost no time for us to relax. With almost no opportunity for us to come down from our fight or flight response, it is no wonder that so many suffer from Anxiety Disorders in one form or another.

But once one begins to realize that work isn't everything, and that one's health is far more important, it may be time to re-prioritize a few things in your life, and to make some necessary lifestyle changes.

Some small changes that could count for a lot include:

- Reducing caffeine
- Avoiding alcohol and nicotine
- Eating a balanced and nutritious diet
- Getting enough sleep
- Regular exercise
- Integrating work-life balance

Herbal Remedies and Supplements

Yes, there are a ton of herbal supplements out there that are always prefaced with the disclaimer that they are not medicine and should not be taken as such, and make no warranties whatsoever as to their effectiveness.

But there is some strong evidence that natural or herbal remedies to have some profound effect. Just make sure to consult your health professional before taking any herbs or nutritional supplements – even if they are labeled "safe," they can still potentially react adversely to any medication you may be taking. Bottom line, don't take any supplements unless approved by your doctor.

Just some of the most popular supplements for Anxiety Disorders include Vitamin B-12, Kava Root, Chamomile Tea,

Valerian, Passionflower, L-theanine, Omega-3 Fatty Acids, St. John's Wort, Inositol, and SAM-e or S-adenosylmethionine supplements.

Acupuncture

This ancient Chinese practice of healing using needles inserted at various crucial points in one's body is said to help unblock the body's energy flow. It is still not considered a part of Western medicine, but evidence of its effectiveness has been pretty much consistent throughout the years.

Self-help Methods for Relieving Anxiety

Try Laughter

We've all heard how laughter is the best medicine, and perhaps no other remedy can be so effective in relieving feelings of anxiety, worry and fear.

Try putting together a laugh kit consisting of joke books or comedy videos that you can dip into when you are feeling down. As an alternative, there are some laughing phone apps now available which you can download on your phone.

Even if you're not feeling particularly humorous and don't really mean your laughter, just getting things going can already help. Laughter stimulates dopamine in the brain, which gives you a hit of reward or pleasure.

Aromatherapy

Various aromatherapy kits have been marketed for their various healing and calming properties. Lavender is just one of the popular scents associated with relaxation.

Aromatherapy can be particularly effective when combined with a massage.

Grounding through tangible activities

For those who are feeling particularly stressed, with myriad and uncontrollable thoughts running through their heads, doing something tangible and very down-to-earth not only helps them relax, it also helps channel all their mental energy to something physical.

Doing housework, cleaning, exercising, etc. These activities are designed to get you out of your head and to focus on something mundane, relaxing, and hopefully, distracting.

Make some time for yourself

If you are bombarded by stress from home, at work, during traffic, etc., maybe you really just need to take some time for yourself. Go on a vacation, get a massage, go to the spa, or other similar retreats can help you recharge, and better yet, get your priorities in order.

Chapter Eight: The Future of Anxiety Disorders

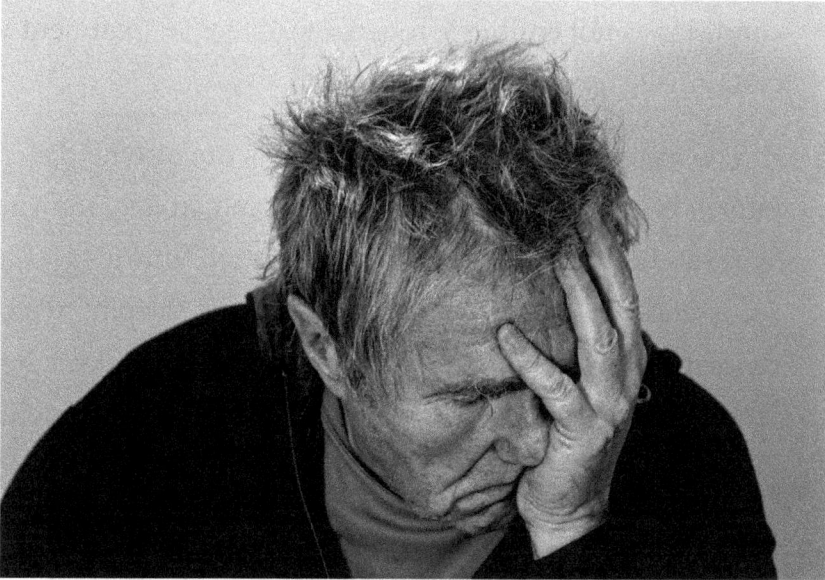

Whether or not a person recovers completely from an Anxiety Disorder, or gains enough coping strategies so that anxiety symptoms are no longer so debilitating, ultimately depend upon each individual circumstance. Various factors come into play: how early the condition was diagnosed and treated, the causes, the severity or degree of the symptoms, and the commitment and response to treatment.

In general, if a condition is caught early, and appropriate treatment given, the outlook of a person suffering from an Anxiety Disorder is good. This is why spreading awareness is important – it simply will not help a child suffering from an Anxiety Disorder if his condition goes unrecognized and untreated until well into his adult years. By then, while the condition is not entirely irreversible, effective treatment will certainly be more difficult.

The introduction of lifestyle changes can also help a person better manage the daily stress and anxiety they may be feeling can go a long way in preventing future recurrences of Anxiety attacks. Eating and sleeping well, reducing one's caffeine, alcohol, and nicotine intake, a better work-balance, and a supportive social and family structure all but helps to guarantee that future episodes of anxiety will no longer be quite so severe.

It probably will not help to tell a person suffering from an Anxiety Disorder that "there is nothing to worry about," but a reassurance that treatment has often proven effective could at least reduce the nervous tension and worry, as well as encourage proactive measures to address attacks of anxiety.

Future Research into Anxiety Disorders

There are exciting new developments in the field of Neuroscience that may help in the better diagnosis and formulation of treatment methods for Anxiety Disorders.

Understanding better how the brain works during a fight or flight response, or during moments of anxiety, can help us better understand this disorder, as well as the expected effects of any prescribed drugs or medication.

Whether you are talking about brain circuitry, measuring chemical or hormonal changes, the role of genetics, or differences in brain activity patterns, understanding how the brain responds during moments of stress, fear or anxiety can help produce better or more targeted treatment methods.

Index

C

D

E

L

M

N

O

P

R

S

T

W

Y

Photo References

Page 1 Photo by suvajit via Pixabay. <https://pixabay.com/en/portrait-dark-light-man-face-dark-915230/>

Page 9 Photo by Wes Washington via Wikimedia Commons. <https://commons.wikimedia.org/wiki/File:Portrait_of_acute _anxiety.JPG>

Page 25 Photo by quinntheislander via Pixabay. <https://pixabay.com/en/traveler-traveller-young-woman-1556516/>

Page 33 Photo by xusenru via Pixabay. <https://pixabay.com/en/portrait-grim-girl-cover-books-1634421/>

Page 43 Photo by johnhain via Pixabay. <https://pixabay.com/en/masks-persona-duality-polarity-827730/>

Page 71 Photo by kheinz via Pixabay. <https://pixabay.com/en/portrait-child-hands-317041/>

Page 77 Photo by tiyowprasetyo via Pixabay. <https://pixabay.com/en/counseling-stress-angry-99740/>

Page 85 Photo by Devanath via Pixabay. <https://pixabay.com/en/oil-rose-aroma-aromatherapy-1205635/>

Page 93 Photo by geralt via Pixabay. <https://pixabay.com/en/despair-alone-being-alone-archetype-513529/>

References

"10 Anxiety Myths Debunked." Madeline R. Vann, MPH. <http://www.everydayhealth.com/anxiety/10-anxiety-myths-debunked.aspx>

"10 Things People Get Wrong About Anxiety." Lindsay Holmes. <http://www.huffingtonpost.com/2014/03/12/anxiety-myths_n_4899290.html>

"12 Signs You May Have an Anxiety Disorder." Amanda MacMillan. <http://www.health.com/health/gallery/0,,20646990,00.html>

"17 Harmful Myths About Anxiety That You Need To Stop Believing." Anna Borges. <https://www.buzzfeed.com/annaborges/anxiety-mythbusters?utm_term=.pqD1EYZLaO#.om0ZJNaE8W>

"6 Cheap, Natural, and Quick Anxiety Remedies."Kathleen Doheny. <http://www.everydayhealth.com/news/cheap-natural-quick-anxiety-remedies/>

"7 Myths About Anxiety Disorder." Caitlin Flynn. <https://www.bustle.com/articles/110773-7-myths-about-anxiety-disorder>

"A Brief History of Anxiety." Calm Clinic.
<http://www.calmclinic.com/brief-history-of-anxiety>

"Agoraphobia." Healthline.
<http://www.healthline.com/health/agoraphobia#Overvi
ew1>

"Agoraphobia." MedlinePlus.
<https://medlineplus.gov/ency/article/000923.htm>

"Agoraphobia." NHS Choices.
<http://www.nhs.uk/Conditions/Agoraphobia/Pages/Intr
oduction.aspx>

"Agoraphobia." Wikipedia.
<https://en.wikipedia.org/wiki/Agoraphobia>

"Agoraphobia: The Fear of Fear." David Carbonell, Ph.D.
<http://www.anxietycoach.com/agoraphobia.html>

"Alternative Treatments for Anxiety." Erica Cirino and the
Healthline Editorial Team.
<http://www.healthline.com/health/anxiety-alternative-
treatments>

"Alternatives for Mood Disorders." Jeanie Lerche Davis.
<http://www.medicinenet.com/script/main/art.asp?article
key=52227>

"Answers to Your Questions about Panic Disorder."
American Psychological Association.
<http://www.apa.org/topics/anxiety/panic-disorder.aspx>

"Anxiety." American Psychological Association.
<http://www.apa.org/topics/anxiety/>

"Anxiety." Wikipedia.
<https://en.wikipedia.org/wiki/Anxiety>

"Anxiety Diagnosis." Healthline.
<http://www.healthline.com/health/anxiety-diagnosis>

"Anxiety Disorder." Wikipedia.
<https://en.wikipedia.org/wiki/Anxiety_disorder>

"Anxiety Disorders." Cleveland Clinic.
<http://my.clevelandclinic.org/health/articles/anxiety-disorders>

"Anxiety Disorders." NAMI. <https://www.nami.org/Learn-More/Mental-Health-Conditions/Anxiety-Disorders>

"Anxiety Disorders." National Institute of Mental Health.
<https://www.nimh.nih.gov/health/topics/anxiety-disorders/index.shtml>

"Anxiety Disorders." University of Maryland Medical Center.

<http://umm.edu/health/medical/reports/articles/anxiety-disorders>

"Anxiety Disorders and Anxiety Attacks." HelpGuide.org. <https://www.helpguide.org/articles/anxiety/anxiety-attacks-and-anxiety-disorders.htm>

"Anxiety Disorders Differential Diagnosis." Nita V Bhatt, MD, MPH. <http://emedicine.medscape.com/article/286227-differential>

"Anxiety Disorders in Children." NHS Choices. <http://www.nhs.uk/conditions/anxiety-children/Pages/Introduction.aspx>

"Anxiety Glossary." Social Anxiety Disorder.net. <http://www.socialanxietydisorder.net/anxiety-glossary>

"Anxiety Glossary of Terms." WebMD. <http://www.emedicinehealth.com/anxiety/glossary_em.htm>

"Anxiety Myths and Misconceptions." Anxietycentre.com. <http://www.anxietycentre.com/anxiety-myths.shtml>

"Anxiety: myths and facts." Charlotte Harding. <http://www.dailymail.co.uk/health/article-131358/Anxiety-myths-facts.html>

"Anxiety Myths & Facts." SFNSW. <https://www.sfnsw.org.au/Mental-Illness/Anxiety/Anxiety-Myths---Facts>

"Anxiety Prognosis." Schizophrenia Fellowship of NSW. <http://www.sfnsw.org.au/Mental-Illness/Anxiety/Anxiety-Prognosis>

"Brain Activity Patterns in Anxiety – Prone People Suggests Deficits in Handling Fear." National Institute of Mental Health. <https://www.nimh.nih.gov/news/science-news/2011/brain-activity-patterns-in-anxiety-prone-people-suggest-deficits-in-handling-fear.shtml>

"Brain Imaging Predicts Psychotherapy Success in Patients with Social Anxiety Disorder." National Institute of Mental Health. <https://www.nimh.nih.gov/news/science-news/2013/brain-imaging-predicts-psychotherapy-success-in-patients-with-social-anxiety-disorder.shtml>

"Children and Teens." ADAA. <https://www.adaa.org/living-with-anxiety/children>

"Childhood Anxiety & Related Disorders." AnxietyBC. <https://www.anxietybc.com/parenting/childhood-anxiety>

"Circuitry for Fearful Feelings, Behavior Untangled in Anxiety Disorders." National Institute of Mental Health. <https://www.nimh.nih.gov/news/science-news/2016/circuitry-for-fearful-feelings-behavior-untangled-in-anxiety-disorders.shtml>

"Common Myths." Selective Mutism Foundation. <https://www.selectivemutismfoundation.org/info-on-selective-mutism/common-myths>

"Complementary & Alternative Treatments." ADAA. <https://www.adaa.org/finding-help/treatment/complementary-alternative-treatment>

"Complementary and Alternative Treatments for Anxiety." Sigal Sharf. <https://www.anxiety.org/complementary-and-alternative-treatments-for-anxiety>

"Description of Child Anxiety Disorders." The Child Anxiety Network. <http://www.childanxiety.net/Anxiety_Disorders.htm>

"GAD." Beyond Blue. <https://www.beyondblue.org.au/the-facts/anxiety/types-of-anxiety/gad>

"Generalized Anxiety Disorder (GAD)." HelpGuide.org. <https://www.helpguide.org/articles/anxiety/generalized-anxiety-disorder-gad.htm>

"Generalized anxiety disorder." Mayo Clinic.
<http://www.mayoclinic.org/diseases-
conditions/generalized-anxiety-
disorder/basics/definition/con-20024562>

"Generalized Anxiety Disorder." WebMD.
<http://www.webmd.com/anxiety-
panic/guide/generalized-anxiety-disorder>

"Generalized anxiety disorder." Wikipedia.
<https://en.wikipedia.org/wiki/Generalized_anxiety_diso
rder>

"Generalized Anxiety Disorder (GAD)." ADAA.
<https://www.adaa.org/understanding-
anxiety/generalized-anxiety-disorder-gad>

"Generalised Anxiety Disorder in Adults – Treatment." NHS
Choices.
<http://www.nhs.uk/Conditions/Anxiety/Pages/Treatme
nt.aspx>

"Generalized Anxiety Disorder: When Worry Gets Out of
Control." NIH.
<https://www.nimh.nih.gov/health/publications/generali
zed-anxiety-disorder-gad/index.shtml>

"Glossary." Child Mind Institute.
<https://childmind.org/topics-a-z/glossary/>

"Glossary of Terms." Canadian Network for Mood and
Anxiety Treatments. <http://www.canmat.org/di-
glossary.php>

"History of Anxiety Disorders." Natasha Tracy.
<http://www.healthyplace.com/anxiety-
panic/articles/history-of-anxiety-disorders/>

"How You Get Diagnosed With Anxiety." CalmClinic.
<http://www.calmclinic.com/anxiety/diagnosis>

"In the Arcadian Woods." George Makari.
<https://opinionator.blogs.nytimes.com/2012/04/16/in-
the-arcadian-woods/>

" "Myth-Conceptions," About Anxiety." ADAA.
<https://www.adaa.org/understanding-anxiety/myth-
conceptions>

"Obsessive-Compulsive Disorder (OCD)." ADAA.
<https://www.adaa.org/understanding-
anxiety/obsessive-compulsive-disorder-ocd>

"Obsessive Compulsive Disorder." AnxietyBC.
<https://www.anxietybc.com/parenting/obsessive-
compulsive-disorder>

"Obsessive Compulsive Disorder (OCD)." Canadian Mental
Health Association.

<http://www.cmha.ca/mental_health/obsessive-compulsive-disorder/#.WJStJF9_fIU>

"Obsessive-Compulsive Disorder (OCD)." Helpguide.org. <https://www.helpguide.org/articles/anxiety/obsessive-compulsive-disorder-ocd.htm>

"Obsessive compulsive disorder (OCD)." Mind. <http://www.mind.org.uk/information-support/types-of-mental-health-problems/obsessive-compulsive-disorder-ocd/#.WJStJl9_fIU>

"Obsessive compulsive disorder (OCD)." NHS Choices. <http://www.nhs.uk/conditions/obsessive-compulsive-disorder/Pages/Introduction.aspx>

"Obsessive-Compulsive Disorder." WebMD. <http://www.webmd.com/mental-health/obsessive-compulsive-disorder#1>

"Panic Attack." Wikipedia. <https://en.wikipedia.org/wiki/Panic_attack#Epidemiology>

"Panic Disorder." Beyond Blue. <https://www.beyondblue.org.au/the-facts/anxiety/types-of-anxiety/panic-disorder>

"Panic Disorder." Darla Burke.
   <http://www.healthline.com/health/panic-
   disorder#Overview1>

"Panic Disorder." NHS Choices. <w
   nhs.uk/conditions/panic-
   disorder/Pages/Introduction.aspx>

"Panic Disorder." WebMD.
   <http://www.webmd.com/anxiety-panic/guide/mental-
   health-panic-disorder>

"Panic Disorder." Wikipedia.
   <https://en.wikipedia.org/wiki/Panic_disorder>

"Panic Disorder & Agoraphobia." ADAA.
   <https://www.adaa.org/understanding-anxiety/panic-
   disorder-agoraphobia>

"Panic Disorder: When Fear Overwhelms." National
   Institute of Mental Health.
   <https://www.nimh.nih.gov/health/publications/panic-
   disorder-when-fear-overwhelms/index.shtml>

"Parenting Tips for Anxious Kids." Worrywisekids.org.
   <http://www.worrywisekids.org/node/36>

"Post-Traumatic Stress Disorder." National Institute of
   Mental Health.

<https://www.nimh.nih.gov/health/topics/post-traumatic-stress-disorder-ptsd/index.shtml>

"Post-Traumatic Stress Disorder (PTSD)." Canadian Mental Health Association. <http://www.cmha.ca/mental_health/post-traumatic-stress-disorder/#.WJTBbF9_fIU>

"Post-traumatic stress disorder (PTSD)." Mind. <http://www.mind.org.uk/information-support/types-of-mental-health-problems/post-traumatic-stress-disorder-ptsd/#.WJTBb19_fIU>

"Post-traumatic stress disorder (PTSD)." NHS Choices. <http://www.nhs.uk/conditions/post-traumatic-stress-disorder/Pages/Introduction.aspx>

"Preventing Anxiety." WebMD. <http://www.webmd.com/anxiety-panic/preventing-anxiety>

"Psychological Treatments for anxiety." Beyond Blue. <https://www.beyondblue.org.au/the-facts/anxiety/treatments-for-anxiety/psychological-treatments-for-anxiety>

"PTSD." Beyond Blue. <https://www.helpguide.org/articles/ptsd-trauma/post-traumatic-stress-disorder.htm>

"PTSD Symptoms, Self-Help, and Treatment."
HelpGuide.org.
<https://www.helpguide.org/articles/ptsd-trauma/post-traumatic-stress-disorder.htm>

"Selective Mutism." American Speech-Language Hearing
Association.
<http://www.asha.org/public/speech/disorders/Selective
Mutism/>

"Selective Mutism." AnxietyBC.
<https://www.anxietybc.com/parenting/selective-mutism>

"Selective Mutism." NHS Choices.
<http://www.nhs.uk/conditions/selective-mutism/Pages/Introduction.aspx>

"Selective Mutism." Wikipedia.
<https://en.wikipedia.org/wiki/Selective_mutism>

"Separation Anxiety." AnxietyBC.
<https://www.anxietybc.com/parenting/separation-anxiety-disorder>

"Separation Anxiety Disorder." Child Anxiety.net.
<http://www.childanxiety.net/Separation_Anxiety.htm>

"Separation Anxiety Disorder." Wikipedia.
<https://en.wikipedia.org/wiki/Separation_anxiety_disor
der>

"Separation Anxiety Disorder Symptoms." Steve Bressert,
Ph.D. <https://psychcentral.com/disorders/separation-
anxiety-disorder-symptoms/>

"Separation Anxiety in Children." HelpGuide.org.
<https://www.helpguide.org/articles/anxiety/separation-
anxiety-in-children.htm>

"Separation Anxiety in Children." WebMD.
<http://www.webmd.com/children/guide/separation-
anxiety#1>

"Social Anxiety and Social Phobia." HelpGuide.org.
<https://www.helpguide.org/articles/anxiety/social-
anxiety-disorder-and-so>cial-phobia.htm>

"Social Anxiety Disorder." ADAA.
<https://www.adaa.org/understanding-anxiety/social-
anxiety-disorder>

"Social Anxiety Disorder." NHS Choices.
<http://www.nhs.uk/conditions/social-
anxiety/Pages/Social-anxiety.aspx>

"Social Anxiety Disorder." Wikipedia.
<https://en.wikipedia.org/wiki/Social_anxiety_disorder>

"Social Anxiety Disorder: More Than Just Shyness."
National Institute of Mental Health.
<https://www.nimh.nih.gov/health/publications/social-anxiety-disorder-more-than-just-shyness/index.shtml>

"Social Anxiety Fact Sheet: What is Social Anxiety Disorder?
Symptoms, Treatment, Prevalence, Medications, Insight,
Prognosis." Social Anxiety Association.
<http://socialphobia.org/social-anxiety-disorder-definition-symptoms-treatment-therapy-medications-insight-prognosis>

"Specific Phobia. Anxiety BC.
<https://www.anxietybc.com/adults/specific-phobia>

"Specific Phobia." Wikipedia.
<https://en.wikipedia.org/wiki/Specific_phobia>

"Specific Phobia Basics." Child Mind Institute.
<https://childmind.org/guide/specific-phobia/>

"Specific Phobias." Beyond Blue.
<https://www.beyondblue.org.au/the-facts/anxiety/types-of-anxiety/specific-phobias

"Specific Phobias." National Institute of Mental Health. <https://www.nimh.nih.gov/health/topics/anxiety-disorders/specific-phobias.shtml>

"Specific Phobias." Perelman School of Medicine University of Pennsylvania. <https://www.med.upenn.edu/ctsa/phobias_symptoms.html>

"Specific Phobias." WebMD. <http://www.webmd.com/anxiety-panic/specific-phobias>

"Symptoms and Causes." Mayo Clinic. <http://www.mayoclinic.org/diseases-conditions/anxiety/symptoms-causes/dxc-20168124>

"Tests and diagnosis." Mayo Clinic Staff. <http://www.mayoclinic.org/diseases-conditions/generalized-anxiety-disorder/basics/tests-diagnosis/con-20024562>

"Tips for Parents and Caregivers." ADAA. <https://www.adaa.org/living-with-anxiety/children/tips-parents-and-caregivers>

"Treating Anxiety Disorders in Children & Adolescents." Cleveland Clinic Children's. <http://my.clevelandclinic.org/childrens-hospital/health-

info/ages-
stages/childhood/hic_Treating_Anxiety_Disorders_in_Ch
ildren_and_Adolescents>

"Treating generalized anxiety Disorder." NHS Choices.
<http://www.nhs.uk/Conditions/Anxiety/Pages/Treatme
nt.aspx>

"Treatment." Anxiety Disorders Association of Canada.
<http://www.anxietycanada.ca/english/treatment.php>

"Treatments for Anxiety." Beyond Blue.
https://www.beyondblue.org.au/the-
facts/anxiety/treatments-for-anxiety>

"What are Anxiety Disorders?" American Psychiatric
Association. <https://www.psychiatry.org/patients-
families/anxiety-disorders/what-are-anxiety-disorders>

"What Are Anxiety Disorders?" WebMD.
<http://www.webmd.com/anxiety-panic/guide/mental-
health-anxiety-disorders>

"What causes anxiety?" Beyond Blue.
<https://www.beyondblue.org.au/the-facts/anxiety/what-
causes-anxiety>

"What is Agoraphobia?" WebMD.
<http://www.webmd.com/anxiety-panic/agoraphobia>

"What is PTSD?" National Center for PTSD.
<https://www.helpguide.org/articles/ptsd-trauma/post-traumatic-stress-disorder.htm>

"What is Selective Mutism?" Selective Mutism Foundation.
<https://www.selectivemutismfoundation.org/info-on-selective-mutism/what-is-selective-mutism>

"What is Social Anxiety?" Social Anxiety Institute.
<https://socialanxietyinstitute.org/what-is-social-anxiety>

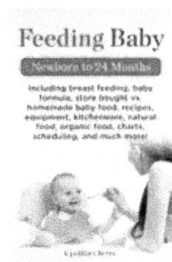

Feeding Baby
Cynthia Cherry
978-1941070000

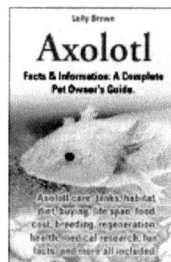

Axolotl
Lolly Brown
978-0989658430

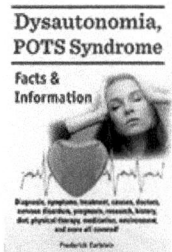

Dysautonomia, POTS
Syndrome
Frederick Earlstein
978-0989658485

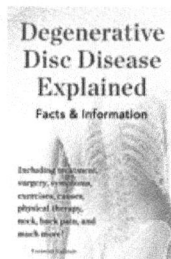

Degenerative Disc
Disease Explained
Frederick Earlstein
978-0989658485

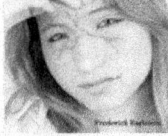

Sinusitis, Hay Fever,
Allergic Rhinitis Explained
Frederick Earlstein
978-1941070024

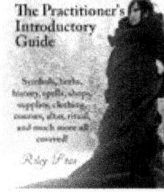

Wicca
Riley Star
978-1941070130

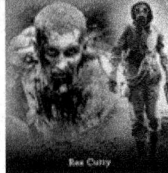

Zombie Apocalypse
Rex Cutty
978-1941070154

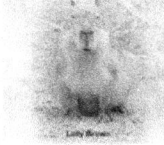

Capybara
Lolly Brown
978-1941070062

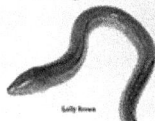

Eels As Pets
Lolly Brown
978-1941070167

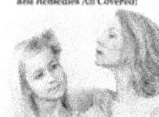

Scabies and Lice Explained
Frederick Earlstein
978-1941070017

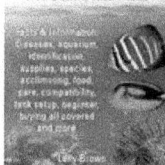

Saltwater Fish As Pets
Lolly Brown
978-0989658461

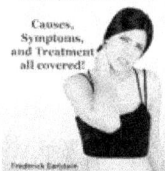

Torticollis Explained
Frederick Earlstein
978-1941070055

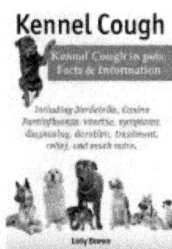

Kennel Cough
Lolly Brown
978-0989658409

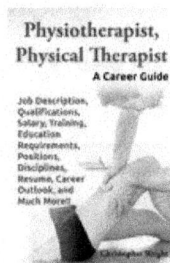

Physiotherapist, Physical
Therapist
Christopher Wright
978-0989658492

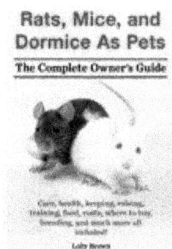

Rats, Mice, and Dormice
As Pets
Lolly Brown
978-1941070079

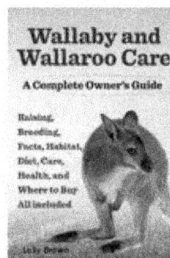

Wallaby and Wallaroo Care
Lolly Brown
978-1941070031

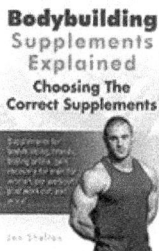

Bodybuilding Supplements
Explained
Jon Shelton
978-1941070239

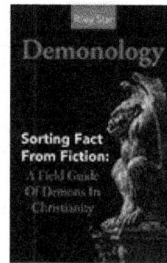

Demonology
Riley Star
978-19401070314

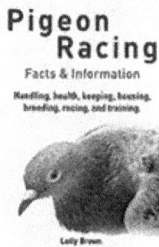

Pigeon Racing
Lolly Brown
978-1941070307

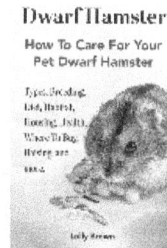

Dwarf Hamster
Lolly Brown
978-1941070390

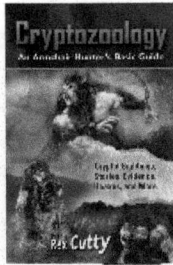

Cryptozoology
Rex Cutty
978-1941070406

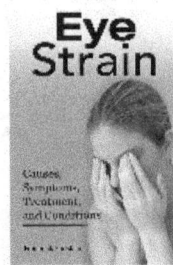

Eye Strain
Frederick Earlstein
978-1941070369

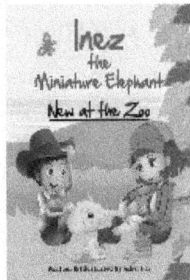

Inez The Miniature Elephant
Asher Ray
978-1941070353

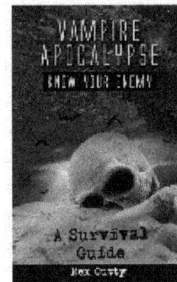

Vampire Apocalypse
Rex Cutty
978-1941070321

www.ingramcontent.com/pod-product-compliance
Lightning Source LLC
Chambersburg PA
CBHW060044210326
41520CB00009B/1261